JACQUES LACAN

the death
of an
intellectual
hero

JACQUES LACAN

the death
of an
intellectual
hero

STUART SCHNEIDERMAN

harvard
university
press

cambridge,
massachusetts
london,
england

1983

Library of Congress Cataloging in Publication Data

Schneiderman, Stuart, 1943–
    Jacques Lacan: the death of an intellectual hero.

    1. Lacan, Jacques, 1901–1981.   2. Psychoanalysts—
France—Biography.   3. Psychoanalysis—France—History—
20th century.   I. Title.
BF109.L28S36   1983   150.19′5′0924   82   21236
ISBN 0-674-47115-6

prologue

I WENT TO PARIS TO BE PSYCHOANALYZED BY JACQUES Lacan. For several years I had labored through his writings, handicapped by an imperfect knowledge of the French language and a basic ignorance of psychoanalytic practice. Despite this, I found in Lacan's work a sense of intellectual excitement and courage that seemed to be lacking in my literary studies.

My previous exploration of literature, especially Shakespeare, had prepared me well to appreciate Lacan. His writings are finely wrought, even overwrought, and they do not easily make sense. In this they resemble poetry, and like poetry they yield to critical thinking. Yet this resemblance is a ploy, a rhetorical ploy. This was my thought when I decided that it would be contradictory for me to continue explicating texts when I knew nothing of the experience from which the texts were drawn. Thus I left Buffalo and a career as professor of English to become a Lacanian psychoanalyst.

My transition, or passage, or translation, is the subject of this book. Rather than offer a critical commentary on Lacan's texts or an elaboration of his theory, I want to re-enact my experience of psychoanalysis with Jacques Lacan, rhetorically.

Lacan lived for eighty tumultuous years and made a very successful career out of saying things that just about no one could understand. He provoked a series of bitter struggles within the world of psychoanalysis, which led in the 1960s to his expulsion from the International Psychoanalytic Association. Deprived of professional recognition and a world stage, Lacan was limited to being outrageous in Paris. He had his own Freudian school there, and among his friends were Maurice Merleau-Ponty, Alberto Giacometti, André Malraux, Roman Jakobson, Claude Lévi-Strauss, Salvador Dali, Pablo Picasso, and Jean-Paul Sartre.

In the mid-sixties general Parisian opinion had it that Lacan was "le seul génie du moment." At the time few took this too seriously; it was only another intellectual fad. The years would prove them wrong. The importance and influence of Lacan deepened, and, within an environment studded with brilliant intellectual stars, his word gained an authority reserved only for the very great. And within the world of psychoanalysis only Freud had the same kind of personal following and respect, to say nothing of the same hostility.

Admittedly, these judgments are debatable. All the more because Lacan's writings are so difficult of access that readers generally can't get enough of a grip on the material to formulate their own judgments. The responsibility for this is necessarily Lacan's. He seems to have gone to great lengths to prevent people from finding out what he had to say. Some have tried to justify this as a teaching device, and a good argument has been made to the effect that this is indeed psychoanalytic. Yet nothing obliges us to follow Lacan through the realm of the abstruse. If his theory has validity, one should be able to articulate it with clarity and precision. This is a task I have set myself.

Still, my decision to write the book was not altogether autonomous. In some sense it was imposed on me by the place I inhabit. That is a fancy way, a Lacanian way, of saying that the form of my book is the result of several years of dialogue about Lacan with American psychoanalysts and intellectuals. Lacan thought that American analysts were irrevocably opposed to him and that his thought could never be accepted in this country. We can't tell whether or not Lacanian theory will be embraced by Americans. On the subject of outright American hostility, Lacan was wrong. My own experience with the American psychoanalytic community has shown me that there is a clear interest in seeking out those places where Lacan made contributions that might help analysts on these shores in their theorization and practice. So I dedicate this book to all of those Americans who have wanted to learn more about Lacan, who have discussed and debated the salient points of theory and practice, and who have often taught me as much about Lacan as I have taught them.

Jacques Lacan died in Paris on September 9, 1981.

1

A WELL-KNOWN LOGICAL PARADOX READS AS FOLLOWS: This statement is false. Would it be equivalent if the first sentence in this book read: This is not the beginning. If the book were a fiction, if I were beginning *in medias res* or anywhere else, the statement would not be paradoxical. But then you might say: That in itself is a paradox, the fact that the statement is not paradoxical.

This book is not an introduction to Lacan. And yet I know full well that I intend to address the book to a general reader, not a specialist in matters psychoanalytic, not a specialist in Lacan, to someone who is simply trying to get a handle on Lacan. Is it a sleight of hand to begin this introduction with the statement: This book is a conclusion. However much I may wish to introduce you to Lacan—a man who was my analyst and mentor—this is now impossible because Lacan is dead. But, then again, I am what is called a Lacanian, and one of the things that means is that maybe I will do it anyway.

When Lacan was alive I published four essays that purported to be introductions. They say something like: Here he is, my old friend Lacan, I want you to meet him; I have profited from knowing him and maybe you will too. Noble sentiments, you may think, decorous, courteous, *comme il faut.* Of these introductions one was published in 1971 in *Diacritics;* one appeared in *Psychology Today* in 1978; and the last two were included in a volume about the school of Lacan that I edited and translated for Yale University Press, entitled *Returning to Freud* (1980). After that I stopped writing introductions, and started asking myself why I stopped. One thought that crossed my mind was that writing introductions, proposing to introduce people to a man who was anything but decorous, is a contradiction in terms. My good intentions were sundered by an internal contradiction. Philippe Sollers, critic, novelist, and a friend of Lacan's, said that Lacan had bad manners—no, not bad, execrable. Now why would I want to introduce you to someone who had execrable manners? Perhaps I am neurotic and want you to share my neurosis?

If I am, you might counsel me a few sessions of psychoanalysis to resolve my inner conflicts. Why not? Of course, Lacan was my analyst and my analysis terminated several years ago. Besides, Lacan is dead, and if I want to return to him to ask him a question, I can only do so through a fiction or a dream. So what would Lacan have said about my abjuring the art of writing introductions? Perhaps it would have gone something like this: "*Cher ami,* the answer is clear, you wrote four introductions and then stopped because you don't know how to count beyond four." Lacan never did address me in those terms, but that is neither here nor there. The statement is characteristic of the way he thought about things; he could have said it. As a matter of fact, during his seminars Lacan sometimes mused about how high his analysands could count.

Now you see that I should have shown some circumspection before trying to introduce you to a man who talked like that. Unless, of course, I had said: This man is a Zen master. On that note I could have made a proper introduction. The problem is that Lacan always insisted on being thought of as a Freudian psychoanalyst. Everyone knows that Freudian psychoanalysts, whatever their quirks, don't talk like that, they don't indulge in quasi-sophistical, narcissistic mumbo-jumbo. If you think you are having a problem with Lacan, just think how the classical and orthodox Freudians felt when Lacan looked at them and said: "Hypocrite lecteur, mon semblable, mon frère."

Actually, to be honest, Lacan never said that to the group of orthodox Freudians called the International Psychoanalytic Association. He might just as well have, for they reacted to him phobically. What is interesting and at the same time Lacanian is that these lies I am inventing tell more about certain situations than truths or facts do.

Before going any further I will tell you that Lacan was wrong: I can count beyond four. This does not make him a bad analyst. As Edward Glover said, there is a therapeutic effect to inexact interpretation. The point is: What did Lacan mean when he spoke of counting up to four? Certainly, he did not mean one, two, three, four, five ... This I have known how to do since the moment I discovered that my fingers were digits. Most people think that such things are trivial, as common sense tells them. And yet most people also learn to count on their fingers, assuming of course that they learn to count, and how is it that these same digits, being identified as one, two, three, four, five, are also my fingers?

If it were merely a question of the fingers on one hand, then I would have no difficulty counting beyond four, up to five. The problem would arise in getting to six. For the sake of argument, let us limit ourselves to the one hand and ask how I get to six. You must remember doing this: you go back to the beginning and recount the same fingers. Thus finger one becomes finger six or else the first digit becomes the sixth digit. Obviously this is another logical problem, because you cannot do arithmetic very well if the first digit and the sixth are the same. And, besides, by now you must think that your psychoanalyzed author has lost his mind. How could anyone justify psychoanalysis and the results of a psychoanalytic treatment when he can arrive at a statement like the following: Someone who has completed a successful psychoanalysis spends his time wondering about the sixth finger on his right hand or whether or not he knows how to count to four. Would it not be better to say that I emerged from my psychoanalysis a whole person, an authentic being, fulfilled and contented, able to work and to love? After all, those are things that everyone wants and strives for through endless analysis or therapy. What kind of nonsense would have it that those things are not the question in analysis and that what we should really concern ourselves about is how someone counting on the fingers of one hand can get to the number six?

In the final analysis, this sounds like Zen. Did you ever try to listen to the sound in "sounds like"? It may be a worthwhile spiritual exercise. It even brings to mind the most famous Zen koan: the sound of the one hand clapping. Now this Zen koan is an enigma; as a matter of fact, it is probably a better riddle than the one about counting to six using one hand. But the point is that the two riddles are the same: if you figure out what the sound of one hand clapping is, then you will know how to count to six with one hand. It is not quite accurate to say that the sound of the one hand clapping is the sixth digit on my right hand, but it is close enough for the moment.

If you read about Zen koans you will know that the correct response to this koan is that the student or novice extends his hand. That is the sound of the one hand clapping. A soundless sound, a name for something that is not. Or better, to use Lacan's term, extending the hand signifies the sound of one hand clapping, soundlessly and also wordlessly. Exemplary instance of what Lacan called "a discourse without words."

In mathematics there is a notation for the sound of the one hand clapping. The set of all the sounds made by one hand clapping is the empty set. The notation is Ø. Now this empty set has a particular function in counting ordinal numbers. The count begins with the empty set and it means that the set of the empty set is one, that is to say, the empty set is written in the brackets that are used in mathematics to designate a set. And you may know that, in order to count to two, you take the set composed of the empty set and the set of the empty set, of 0 and 1, if you like. When Lacan talked about how high people could count, he was talking about the kind of counting that takes place in these terms. And it is no simple matter to keep going this way: three is the set comprising the empty set, the set of the empty set, and the set comprising the empty set and the set of the empty set. At the very least this shows that mathematics would not have advanced too far if it had had to use words. This will not prevent me from showing you that I know how to count to four: four is the set comprising the empty set, the set of the empty set, the set comprising the empty set and the set of the empty set, and the set comprising the empty set and the set of the empty set and the set comprising the empty set and the set of the empty set. Thus, counting up to four is no mean feat. Five is simply the set comprising all the sets designating 0, 1, 2, 3, 4. Note also in this formulation how important the punctuation is: the brackets in set theory and in logic function as punctuation, and as soon as things get a little complicated, they become essential if we are to find our way.

I will spare you the count up to six. From what I have said up to now, the sound of the one hand clapping is not the sixth finger on the one hand; it is the empty set without which we could not count at all in ordinal arithmetic. Once its principle is established, we can count on and on, if we so choose.

Is this simply a sterile exercise, lacking in the marrow of

human emotion? Why would Lacan, a man who wanted to effect psychoanalytic cures, spend his time with subjects that are manifestly outside his field? Or, here is a better question, what are the psychoanalytic versions of these numbers, given that numbers are important in psychoanalysis and also that analysis tends irreducibly to retain some content: analysis cannot be entirely formalized, Lacan said.

In Lacan's theory the empty set has more than one manifestation: what comes to mind most immediately is the empty grave, the empty tomb. I believe Anthony Wilden to have been the first to accent its importance in *The Language of the Self*. The empty grave is important not because of its relationship to death, considered here as a fact of nature, but rather because of its symbolization of the place against which we have to confront the dead. If the dead were at home in their graves, then they would be buried, classed, and we would be finished with them. If the grave is empty, we have to deal with them. The empty grave has a significant role in the story of Christ as well as in that of Hamlet—the appearance of the ghost suggests to Hamlet that the grave has been opened and emptied. Also, there are two central figures in Freudian theory who are noteworthy for not having been buried, for having disappeared without a trace: Oedipus and Moses. (Admittedly, the descendants of Theseus know the site of the grave of Oedipus, but this does not obviate the fact that when Oedipus dies, the place of his grave is unmarked; he disappears. This is a way of signifying the empty set, of marking it with a sign, a sign that is kept secret and is passed down from father to son.)

What then is the set of the empty set? In Lacan's theory this can only be the signifier as one, as singular. We can also say that it is the singular subject, though the subject is not singular unless the signifier as one establishes the concept of oneness. This signifier may be a ghost, or the secret that is kept by the descendants of Theseus, but it is preeminently for Lacan the proper name. The problem we will see later is that the empty grave is also a subject; so the human subject is always split between a mark and a void.

Am I then saying that the theory of psychoanalysis can be constructed out of the empty grave and the signifier? Yes. But, you might object, if this is what Lacan was up to, then he certainly deviated from Freud. These were not Freud's terms, as an examination of the Freudian text establishes beyond doubt. My answer is to recommend that you not be too hasty in drawing a conclusion here, in dismissing Lacan's argument before you know what it is. I would suggest that you look at photographs of Freud's office and note with care the staggering number of funerary objects, objects dug up from the earth by archaeologists. Freud was passionately involved with the process of emptying the earth of human artifacts. He hoarded them himself to such an extent that his offices almost resemble a tomb. And why shouldn't we consider this to be a text in the same way we consider Freud's writings to be a text?

I will not pursue this argument any further for the moment. This book, the one you have in your hands, is designed to demonstrate these points. For the moment we have the elements we need to count, and we can look in a different way at some of the numbers that appear habitually in Freud. I have said that the empty set, whose name is zero, corresponds to the empty grave. I could also have said that it represents the mother's lack of a phallus, a discovery that Freud considered crucial for development. The set of the empty set is the signifier, but why not also see in it the phallic function, so important for Freud and Lacan? The number two appears commonly in psychoanalytic theory as the ego and its object, as me and you, as mother and child, and even in the obsession some people have with dividing the world into inner and outer. Three was one of Lacan's favored numbers; it refers to the triangulation of the Oedipus complex in Freud, and Lacan used it in theorizing the imaginary, real, and symbolic orders, and the Borromean knot. The number four is perhaps the trickiest, but remember that Freud declared once that there are four people involved in every sex act. Lacan has a number of instances where the number four is in play: the schema for intersubjectivity says that there are subject, ego, object, and Other, and a later theorization shows discourse being formed by the movement of four fundamental terms, two signifiers (because at least two are necessary for any signifier to make sense), a barred subject (perhaps this is another representation of the empty grave), and an object called the object *a* (a trace or remainder, as in the Freudian memory trace).

Let us pause here and survey the ground we have covered. What I have been doing in a somewhat circumspect fashion is introducing some of the basic reasoning behind Lacan's theory of psychoanalysis. Remember that extending your hand as the response to the Zen koan of the sound of the one hand clapping also resembles a gesture of introduction: Please allow me to introduce myself . . . But I also said that this book is not an introduction; it is a conclusion. And if you know a little about Zen, you know that the extending of one hand is *not* a gesture of introduction. The novice or candidate must study Zen for years before he gains enough knowledge to respond to the koan. The gesture of introduction is in fact the conclusion of a long process of spiritual discipline, a spiritual ascesis, as Lacan would have called it.

So I have set about to write this conclusion because Lacan's grave is empty. In common parlance this suggests that he has not been properly mourned. In order to be mourned properly Lacan has to be recognized, and we know that he suffered from lack of recognition throughout his life. At least he thought so. He said he was one of those people who will be better recognized after death. This means that Lacan as a living human being was too much of a distraction to people, that the man provoked passions too violent to permit the intellectual activity that can lead to recognition. I would add that Lacan's death intensified the passion of his followers. Thus I am obliged to talk about the man, about the passions that followed him to the grave, and beyond it.

Now, you might ask, by what right do I presume to talk about Lacan the man? Isn't this indiscreet gossip-mongering? Not if I knew the man and thus can write of my own experience with him. This in its turn may lead to the following objection: Since you were in analysis with Lacan, how could you know the man? All of your experiences are only projections on the blank surface that the analyst presented to you. If we know anything about the transference, we know that it is a fundamental falsification of human experience.

In normal circumstances and according to psychoanalytic common sense, this would be a valid objection. With Lacan, though, there are no normal circumstances, and common sense, psychoanalytic or otherwise, is thoroughly unreliable. One of my own peculiar habits of thought tells me this: if everyone believes that an analysand knows very little about his analyst, then that analysand probably knows his analyst rather well, perhaps even better than the analyst's own friends and relations. Most people think that the knowing resides with the analyst, that the analyst knows a lot about his patient. Some people even believe that this disparity in knowledge works to the analyst's advantage, permitting him to exercise power over his patient. To counter these beliefs, Lacan quoted Socrates to the effect that the analyst knows nothing except Eros. If the comparison is germane, the analyst's skill consists in helping someone else to find out what he knows. And we should not fail to note that this last sentence is grammatically equivocal: is the *he* in "he knows" the analyst or the analysand? We can say that it is both: the analysand will discover what he himself knows, but he may well think that this knowledge resides with the analyst. He may therefore be led to ferret out that knowledge or to try to induce the analyst to tell him, or else to read the analyst's words and gestures for clues to the knowledge the analyst retains.

As a general rule, and Lacan was no exception, analysts do not reveal their personalities or feelings, their opinions or biographies, to their analysands. They rarely talk about themselves, and even more rarely will they take a patient into their confidence. The mistake we tend to make, and Lacan was at pains to correct it, is in thinking that when we know about someone this means that we know their life history, their personality, their feelings and emotions. Lacan's view was that all of the above is merely camouflage or persiflage, a buffer that permits people to enter the commerce of everyday life without tearing each other apart.

There are ways of fine-tuning the personality to make the human being more agreeable, more palatable, in human society. Combine these with what is called standing in the community and one arrives at the ideal of respectability. So far as I can tell, in America analysts are deeply concerned with their respectability. Europeans never cease harping on the fact that America is a puritanical country where respectability counts for too much. One would be hard pressed, however, to say that the French are any less concerned with respectability; a country that is still infatuated with aristocracy must retain some notions, and rather precise ones at that, about how to behave in polite society. Good manners and the other accoutrements of social interaction are codified in France at a level that would be beyond the imagination of most Americans. In this atmosphere Lacan was not a respectable man; as the British would put it, he didn't care a fig for respectability. Perhaps Lacan was too enamoured with his role of *enfant terrible* of the psychoanalytic world; perhaps he cherished unduly the position of the heretic or renegade. Whatever the reason, Lacan did not seek respectability—he sought respect. And he received it: not for his pleasant personality, not because he was such a good fellow, not because he was so easy to get along with, but rather because people were in awe of him and approached him with a mixture of fear and reverence. This quality was present to every analysand who walked through the door of his office at 5 rue de Lille.

The Doctor, as he was called respectfully, or the Old Man, as he was called somewhat less respectfully, did not think that psychoanalysis was a respectable profession; he judged it to be a subversive and revolutionary occupation. One day at his seminar Lacan was trying to explain his impenetrable prose style: if they knew what I was saying, he offered, they would never have let me say it. This has a slightly paranoid tinge, but that does not mean he was wrong.

You do not have to be fully conversant with the ways and means of the American psychoanalytic establishment, the orthodox Freudians, I mean, to know that Lacan's constant defiance of respectability did not endear him to them. My impression is that the New York Psychoanalytic Institute, the center of American Freudianism, contains some of the most respectable people I have ever met. That, however, is only half the story. I must also tell you that on one occasion I got the impression that there is a darker side to the respectability of the NYPI. Several years ago I attended a meeting of the society that comprises this institute. This meeting was in honor of Edith Jacobson, eminent psychoanalyst who had just retired. After the usual encomiums and a fine talk by Otto Kernberg, the time came for everyone to adjourn to another room for champagne and cookies. Before the assembled respectable analysts could move from their seats, the master of ceremonies took the microphone to ask them if they would please remain seated until Dr. Jacobson had time to traverse the auditorium and the corridor and was settled in the room containing the champagne and cookies. The m.c. averred that, in their enthusiasm for the refreshments across the hall, the assembled respectable analysts might trample poor Dr. Jacobson, thus abbreviating her retirement.

Now, on the other side of the Atlantic, Lacan had managed to create a reputation for being strange, bizarre, insolent, and at times outrageous. He was prone to making scenes in public, to being abrupt and rude, to expressing his amorous intentions toward women in flagrant ways. (Once, it is told, a taxi driver was so impressed by a love scene between Lacan and a woman in the back seat of his cab that he called for an appointment the next morning and went on to spend several years in analysis with Lacan.) Some of Lacan's behavior would have been more acceptable had he not been a psychoanalyst, and had people not believed that analysts should conform to some ideal of adult behavior. Some of it could have been explained away analytically, though this was hardly Lacan's own approach. Analysis cannot explain everything, and there are flaws of character that do not admit of explanation, and should not. It would be unfair not to note that Lacan was also known as an extremely generous man, that he often showed a degree of hospitality quite out of character in his city, that his devotion and dedication to his patients had few limits. Lacan was often accused of being too intellectual in his theory, in not giving enough play to emotion and affect. It is no small irony that many of those who preached the virtues of affect were the first to condemn Lacan for acting emotionally, for exposing his affects.

It is one thing for Lacan to have had "it," as we say, another for him to have known that he had it, still worse for him to have flaunted it. He never let others forget that he had it; whatever the "it" was. The Lacan mystique, the aura that surrounded him, was based on this "it"; those who accepted Lacan sought his favor because they believed that he would give some of "it" to them, or that they could bask in the afterglow. And certainly many did; being a Lacanian in the glory days of French psychoanalysis, during the mid-seventies, was a ticket to success. Lacan's comment on this was that people who have it do not give it away; this "it" is something that can only be taken from them, and not without a fight.

There are some who say that Lacan's conduct of his life

was the major issue in his exclusion from the International Psychoanalytic Association. Of course there were important theoretical issues in question, especially concerning Lacan's attacks on the theory of ego psychology and his practice of the short session. But the crux of the issue seemed to be the sentiments of Marie Bonaparte, who at first sided with Lacan and his group and who later turned against them to side with the group led by Sacha Nacht. The groups were divided over questions of who was to teach what. But the deciding factor in Lacan's exclusion was the about-face of the Princess, as Marie Bonaparte was called. Wild rumors circulated that Lacan had made a pass at Mme Bonaparte; other more lucid wits answered that her reaction could only be explained by the absence of any such pass. Lacan, though, attributed her behavior to the fact that, when he drew up the by-laws for a new institute, he neglected to give her an honorary position and title in the organization. He felt that this gesture of disrespect had drawn her wrath. Teaming up with the Princess was none other than Anna Freud, and during the discussions held by the executive committee of the IPA the opinion of these two *grandes dames* held sway.

A keen observer of these things, Philippe Sollers, told me that Lacan was expelled because he had run afoul of the matriarchy. How does one go about running afoul of a matriarchy? In the words of Anna Freud, Lacan washed his dirty linen in public. After respectability, the second most important characteristic for a psychoanalyst is discretion, and Lacan was notoriously indiscreet. Conflicts in the world of psychoanalysis in Paris did not stay within this world; they became public events. By the time Lacan had become a "national monument," the splits in the world of French analysis were major news events.

And Lacan's indiscretion was not limited to psychoanalytic affairs; there were whisperings that Lacan was involved in other kinds of affairs, and that he did not limit these to furtive dalliances. Rumor had it that his mistresses were almost as legion his followers. The matriarchs do not much mind these manifestations of masculine libido; they do mind when they are not permitted to ignore them. If these rumors are true, and I am sure that future biographers will find out all there is to know about them and more, then the cardinal sin is not washing one's dirty linen, but dirtying it in public.

Assuming that Lacan's personal behavior was repugnant to certain members of the International Psychoanalytic Association, the conduct of his life did not in France constitute an offense to public morals. If we want to discuss the matter at the level of the affairs of the psychoanalytic institute, there is a good argument to be made for not conducting the operations of such organizations in total clandestinity. Also, the way the politics of such an association is conducted must reflect the politics of the country in which it is anchored. Parisian mores and morals were not always consonant with those of the Anglo-Saxon and Germanic countries in which psychoanalysis had begun and prospered.

Be all this as it may, there was a conflict between the Parisians and the rest of the international group. The source of this conflict may well lie in a difference of cultural traditions. The psychoanalytic movement is heavily Jewish in its inspiration, to say nothing of its membership. Lacan was raised a Catholic; he did not practice Catholicism, but he was educated by Jesuits and his theorizing bears the stamp of his own cultural heritage. Then, too, as against Austria, Germany, Britain, and America, France was a Romance-language country. May we not say that certain habits of thought and social customs, even ethical principles, are linked to different religious, cultural, and linguistic backgrounds? Even today the places where Lacanian thought has been most thoroughly accepted are Italy and South America. The Germans, British, and North Americans find it all to be written in a foreign language, with alien thought patterns. This is not to say that Lacan suffered unusual discrimination because of his culture. But the foreignness of Lacan, the difficulties of his theory and his techniques, as well as his personal behavior, were partly the result of significant cultural differences.

Lacan was excluded, expelled, finally excommunicated by the International; his teaching was denounced, condemned, even cursed to sterility. The IPA would permit him in 1963 to practice analysis, but not to teach or to train candidates. Thus stigmatized, Lacan became a hero to many people whose political opinions placed them in opposition to everything American. Unwittingly the International had laid the groundwork for the fashioning of a legend.

Eventually, everything that Lacan did or said appeared larger than life; he was magnified and scrutinized until he had become almost a monstrosity. In fact, Lacan was larger than life, highly visible to the public, to his public: his every word was taken down on tape, his every gesture studied and analyzed by the many he had influenced. He was not an analyst just like the others; he was an aristocrat, even a tyrant, possessing a theoretical mind the likes of which the psychoanalytic world had not seen since Freud. As I have implied, some of those who had known Freud well did not want to see another mind like his.

There is always considerable difficulty in encountering things that have this quality of strangeness or Otherness. When we do, we often have recourse to one of the intellectual quirks of our age, one of the habits of thought that characterize what Lacan liked to call the "ambient debility": we make a diagnosis. In Paris some people thought that Lacan was a paranoiac; others classed him as schizophrenic or homosexual. Americans are not quite so incontinent and they say that Lacan had a grandiose self, an advanced narcissistic personality disorder, or faulty object relations. At one point speculation in Paris was so rife that Lacan stepped forth to tell the truth. The truth, he said, was that he was a perfect hysteric; he added that a perfect hysteric is one without symptoms.

If Lacan was right, it is a waste of time to attempt to categorize him within the system of psychiatric classification. We know that this system has its faults and that, fine-tune it as we may, there are certain things that must fall outside of the realm of the psychopathological. When I say this I am not referring to normality. From a Lacanian perspective, normality is the apotheosis of psychopathology, since it is basically incurable.

Lacan was decidedly and defiantly not normal: he was bizarre, an odd figure, something like the number three. Nor was he perfect; the perfection of the perfect hysteric is highly imperfect. He would have liked to have been a saint but said that he had no hopes of achieving that goal. Sainthood would have been an ethical perfection. For Lacan, beyond psychopathology lay ethics.

If we renounce finding a symptom or syndrome, what can we say about Lacan the man? We want to read him, not to classify him or to explain him away as the result of not-good-enough mothering. Changing the frame of reference, one can say that Lacan had a flaw, a tragic flaw in the Aristotelian sense. This has the advantage of placing things in the theater; the only way to talk about a perfect hysteric is theatrically. Not everyone, of course, lives his life histrionically. Some people think that life is a laboratory experiment; some that it is a classroom or learning experience, some that it is a history book or a sociological survey. For Lacan the way that was closest to psychoanalysis was hysteria, in a theatrical mode. What was Lacan's flaw? I see no purpose for looking for something obscure here: his flaw was hubris, and hubris has nothing to do with what is now called the grandiose self.

There was a time when I compared Lacan to Proust's Duchess of Guermantes, a comparison that Lacan did not find wholly displeasing. But this was before I got to Paris. Once I got there in 1973 I changed my mind and decided that Lacan reminded me of King Lear. Certainly Lacan was no Hamlet, procrastinating, doubting, tortured by narcissism and guilt. Lacan's was a tragedy of ingratitude, a play where the only true encounter with the real, with the elements, the storm, takes place as a tragedy. As Lacan said, *King Lear* shows us that when man sets off on the path of his desire, he goes forth alone and betrayed. Anyone who finds himself cast in the role of Lear will not think that destiny is very benevolent. Nor are there many ways out. Lacan's penchant was to accept destiny and to play the role to the hilt. And yet he did try to transform his role, though without total success.

If there is any transformation of Lear, then things are not quite so bleak as they appear at first. Within the world of Shakespearean theater, the obvious transformation is Prospero. In order to become Prospero you are obliged to abjure your art, to break your staff, and to drown your book. When I was in Paris, from 1973 through 1977, I and some of my friends thought that Lacan was the type of man who would not retire gracefully, who would not let himself be put out to pasture. For all intents and purposes this is what happened. The stories that come to us of how it was in his practice and seminar lectures during the last two years are not pretty; nor are they finally acceptable professionally. Lacan was ill at the time and spent long minutes at his seminar staring into space or at the blackboard; there were times when he was not well enough to receive patients. From a brief meeting I had with him in 1979, I got the impression that he was lacking the presence of mind and concentration I had known before. And yet he continued to work through July 1981. Some writers light on this period of his life to discredit him—but I choose to read it as the last act of Lacan's tragedy.

When Prospero retires, abjuring his art, breaking his staff, drowning his book, he is saying that there is no succession.

Whatever he had as a great man cannot be transmitted to others. Prospero thus forestalls the possibility of a war of succession, and in this we have to say he was successful. Lear attempted halfheartedly to retire, attempted to forestall such a war, and was a conspicuous failure at both. When I say that Lacan never succeeded in becoming Prospero, I mean that for the last few years the world of Parisian psychoanalysis has been wracked and perhaps even wrecked by wars of succession. These led from conflict to dissolution to disintegration. When the remains of Lacan's group divided into three warring factions in 1981, the rhetoric was so poisonous, so undisguised in its virulence, that it was thoroughly reminiscent of the discourse of Goneril and Regan. Lacan's truest and most loyal supporters were the youngest of his three daughters and her husband.

Lacan's tragedy was lived out in public. One could argue that Lacan simply wanted recognition, that he expected those who were trained and taught by him to recognize their debt to him. And when they did not, when they showed themselves unequal to their charge, Lacan and the Lacanians lashed out at them, treating them as ingrates, and traitors. Whatever the status of Lacan's desire for recognition, he was an extremely demanding man, of others as of himself. Those whose habits of thought or practice tended to the simple and the superficial, those who refused to confront the difficult questions, those who sought the comfort of confronting petty issues, Lacan had no use for them and never failed to express his disdain. At the height of the analytic debate during 1981 Lacan wrote a letter calling on people to be either with him or against him—those who were not with him were necessarily against him—and demanding nothing less than love. As he had written many years before, all demands are ultimately demands for love. And on the one occasion when Lacan appeared on television, he said that he would not alter his notoriously impenetrable style because he simply did not care to speak to idiots: my discourse, he said, is for those who are not idiots. Accusations of imbecility and the like flowed from Lacan as naturally as water flows downstream. People were afraid of Lacan, afraid of his power: psychoanalysts kowtowed to him or rejected him entirely. And when he was visibly diminished, when he could no longer stand up in public to denounce traitors, those he had trained turned against him as if to right past wrongs. An accumulation of insult and injury, of forced deference, gave way to violent and vengeful attacks. In part these were directed against Lacan, but the brunt of the violence was directed against Lacan's son-in-law, Jacques-Alain Miller, in an exemplary instance of scapegoating. And this did not derive from respect so much as it did from fear, fear of what Lacan once dead might still be able to do. We think we can negotiate with the living; the dead, existing in otherness, are far more difficult to handle.

Whitehead said that the history of philosophy is a series of footnotes to Plato. Before Lacan, the history of psychoanalysis was a series of footnotes to Freud. What is striking about Freud's theoretical production is that it was so far above the rest that the entire theory of psychoanalysis seemed to be the work of one man. It was not as if the theory of dreams were constructed bit by bit through the labors of a team of scientists; the theory of dreams is contained in one book written by one man. In Lacan's France all of the great theoretical constructions were also the work of one man. It is rare that such things should happen. And it is probably true in fields other than psychoanalysis that the place of that one man is unbearable. To be the focal point of a radical break in the fabric of intellectual and cultural history is simply beyond the capacity of any one human being. Anyone who is in this position and who knows it will suffer from hubris.

Lacan was too much for his world and, since that world could not accommodate itself to him, it split apart. Undoubtedly it would have done so no matter what Lacan himself did; his wont was to help it along. Again this is consonant with a tragic perspective, for if in a tragedy there is a clearly defined way for the hero to avoid destruction and if he chooses not to follow it, then he is a fool and not a tragic hero. If a tragedy is to be effective, it must be inexorable. The tragic hero is often one who precipitates the fated conclusion, with full knowledge of what that conclusion will be.

In Lacan's Paris there was a general consensus that the problem was Lacan himself, and if the analysts could have the theory without the man, then all would be well. Everyone would have loved to have the theory without the theorist—clearly an infantile wish. Still this idea had a great hold on people in the analytic world of France, and at the time of his death Lacan had been abandoned or denounced by the majority of those he had trained and who owed him more than just their careers. His death was one of the most anxiously awaited events in recent Parisian intellectual history, and not just within the psychoanalytic group. Lacan had made psychoanalysis into the dominant intellectual discipline in France, and the turmoil and turbulence of the world of Lacan was regularly reported in the French press. The drama surrounding Lacan's dying was played out in public while the exact nature of his illness, even the fact that he was ill, remained one of the best kept secrets in the city.

Analysts in France knew that the death of Lacan would mark the end of an era, the end of the golden age of French analysis. In this they were right. They ought to have known that efforts to make analysis into a science or into a system of knowledge abstracted as pure theory are doomed to failure. The key to interest in psychoanalysis is its connection with the truth of desire. This is palpable, present in psychoanalytic treatment, but it is also present in the surrounding ambiance, the cultural and social atmosphere that supports the treatment. How many people in France became interested in psychoanalysis because of Lacan the man; how many went to his seminars just to see him, in the flesh? Far more than could reasonably be expected to have any understanding of his theories. And I would even suggest that the imperfections of the man, his eccentricity, were precisely what showed people that he had some grasp of truth. Aside from trying to force analysis into the mold of science, the surest way to defeat it is to make its great men into *papier mâché* images of the joys of a normal life. To promote this as a public image, to censor the aspects that are unpleasant or wild, is to make analysis into a rote exercise inspiring only indifference.

When Lacan died on September 9, 1981, the event was an anticlimax. Perhaps because of a process that Robert Jay Lifton calls psychic numbing, people did not seem capable of mustering any true reaction. One analyst told me that Lacan was not mourned significantly because, as he put it, "we did that last year." Others barely noticed his passing because they had come to believe that his soul had taken up habitation in his son-in-law, Jacques-Alain Miller.

At times it seemed that a good number of people were wishing for Lacan's death. There are enough analysts who are still proud of having an Oedipus complex for these scenes to be enacted in Oedipal garb. But the events themselves and Lacan's acts within this world, his world, suggest another reading.

In 1979 a group of dissidents had formed within the Ecole freudienne de Paris whose purpose was to remove Lacan as director not through any Brutus-like act but rather through the judicial process. Lacan reacted in early January 1980 by dissolving the Ecole by fiat. For the record Lacan had no legal right to do such a thing; the by-laws of the association stipulated that a dissolution could take place only through a vote of two thirds of the members. It happened that after nine months of negotiation, haggling, and judicial maneuvering, the two-thirds majority was attained. But that is not the point.

What these events showed was first how little use Lacan had for such things as institutional by-laws. Often enough he broke the rules and set up his own, which then became the rules of others. Lacan was in fact always true to his own rules, which were neither capricious nor arbitrary. They were based on a Law that cannot be comprised by rules of civilized behavior, but that determines desire as the basis for action. This is the only path to the overcoming of narcissism, because desire is always the desire of the Other, as he put it, and because desire always seeks recognition by the Other's desire.

In dissolving the Ecole freudienne, Lacan put an end to the Oedipal psychodrama that some people wanted to stage. Thus he deprived many people of their thoughts about wishing for his death, thereby to replace him. You probably know that people entertain these wishes for the death of a father figure in order to gain certain spoils, namely the woman or women connected to the father figure. When they have these fantasies, they often become wracked with guilt. What is not so well appreciated is the fact that these same people gain a specific satisfaction from this guilt, and they do so narcissistically. In our time guilt is one of the predominant spoils of the Oedipus complex.

To those who wanted to supplant him Lacan was saying that, yes, he was going to die, not because they were strong enough to murder him, but rather that he was going to die because he wanted to. This is the significance of the fact that during his last two or so years Lacan was mostly silent, rarely participating in the storm he had stirred up when he dissolved his school. The refusal to confirm the Oedipus complex as the summit of human development is intrinsically disturbing: one last time Lacan hit his faithful where it hurt; some of them have still not recovered.

The theme of the desire for death is clear and unmistakable in Lacan's work. It organizes the third section of his essay "Function and Field of Speech and Language." This section opens with a quotation concerning the Cumaean Sibyl, condemned to hang in a jar by her hair for a number of years equal to the number of grains of sand on the beach. Some boys come up to her and ask: What do you want? Her answer is: I want to die.

In a speech at a psychoanalytic congress in 1973 Lacan debunked the idea that people are apprehensive about dying. People are more apprehensive about living too long, he said. There are some who believe that Socrates was asked to choose between death and ostracism, and that he chose death because he believed in philosophy. But if you read the *Phaedo*, admittedly a Platonic distortion, you will find veiled in the text the idea that Socrates died because he wanted to, and not because he loved us or Plato or wisdom. At the end of the dialogue Crito suggests that Socrates wait a little longer before taking the poison. Socrates rejects this idea: "I should make myself ridiculous in my own eyes if I clung to life and spared it, when there is no more profit in it."

Lacan died of postoperative complications after a tumor was removed from his intestines. Specifically, his kidneys failed, he lapsed into a coma, and he died. This is true but insufficient; it does not tell us anything about Lacan's removing himself from the operations of the psychoanalytic institute he had founded, his passing the staff, as it appeared, to his son-in-law, Jacques-Alain Miller, his refusal to speak, in public or in private, or to intervene actively. These facts, which are facts as much as a medical report, signify a desire to die. And they do so even if Lacan did not repeat Freud's example of asking his physician to administer a fatal dose of one drug or another. Whatever the illness, all physicians know that the patient's desire to live or to die is often a decisive factor in the success of treatment.

I want to be clear about one central point: the desire to die does not translate into suicide. If, as Lacan put it, one ought to sustain desire and not seek an object that will gratify it and thereby erase it, the desire to die is best enacted when death is kept at a distance. And yet this desire will also know that there is a point beyond which one is simply procrastinating, postponing the inevitable out of fear and anxiety, and at that point one ought to submit. Lear did not die of wanting to die, he resisted to the end, and Freud's reading of the play in his "The Theme of the Three Caskets" states that its truth is the submission to death.

On the other hand, suicide does not represent a desire for death, but rather a love of death. Love is far more impatient than desire; love demands love unconditionally and instantaneously; it demands what is commonly called instant gratification. People who commit suicide are lovers of death, and suicide is an act of love. There are many reasons behind suicide, but one of the most common is the failure of love, its betrayal. Not so much the fact that the one person who was beloved has been lost, but the idea that love itself may have gone also. That there is no more love in the world—this leads to suicide as a last, desperate act of love, an act that may succeed where love has failed between people. He or she may not requite my love, but there is still the hope that death loves me, that death will receive my sacrifice of myself. These acts are often committed by the young, by adolescents, by people for whom love has a far greater meaning than for those who have experienced more of life. And these acts represent a radical refusal to set forth on the path of desire, an inability to tolerate frustration and loss, an inability to defer the encounter with death. There are times when the person who will commit suicide will await the right moment: this is not because he has realized his desire for death, but rather because he wants to assure the success of his act, the acceptability of his offering. Among the finer expressions of the dynamic of suicide is Faulkner's description of Quentin Compson III in the appendix to *The Sound and the Fury*, "who loved death above all, who loved only death, loved and lived in a deliberate and almost perverted anticipation of death as a lover loves and deliberately refrains from the waiting willing friendly tender incredible body of his beloved, until he can no longer bear not the refraining but the restraint and so flings, hurls himself, relinquishing, drowning."

The suicidal act counterpoints the desire for death. As Lacan pointed out, the road to suicide leads through primrose visions of the perfection of love, through the folly of staking everything on hope for tomorrow, on what the French call "les lendemains qui chantent."

2

IT WOULD BE DISINGENUOUS ON MY PART TO TELL ABOUT the life of Lacan when what incited me to write this book was Lacan's death. A man's death has often led some people to attempt to reconstruct a life, to put the pieces of the puzzle together for whatever reason seems to speak to the biographer. This book is a reminiscence; it is not designed to bring Lacan back to life but to assure that his rest will be peaceful.

A reminiscence is a first-person narrative, unabashedly. So to begin at the beginning is to take the moment I arrived in Paris to start my training analysis with Lacan. My arrival in Paris was not what one would call a momentous event. It is no sense of false modesty that prevents me from comparing it to the arrival of Augustine in Carthage. That said, Augustine's decription of his arrival is worth quoting: "To Carthage I came, where a cauldron of unholy loves bubbled up all around me. I loved not as yet, yet I loved to love; and, with a hidden want, I abhorred myself that I wanted not." Whether or not this has anything to do with me, it is as good a Lacanian definition of neurosis as I have ever read.

So, not only was my arrival in Paris in 1973 not momentous, it was for some people slightly bizarre. I had the distinction of being the only American to train with Lacan. I can't say that I found it particularly strange that I arrived in Paris to do what I had set out to do, but being the sole citizen of my country to do so, my presence posed questions in the minds of many people. I should mention that there was another American, a woman, who had trained with Lacan just before I arrived, but she had become a French citizen, and it was perhaps for that reason that Lacan insisted that she was not an American.

The events I am going to recount are a part of my experience and I must recount them as I saw and understood them. And yet I was as much a witness as a participant, an outside observer, and it is not evident that the confidences that people make to an American in Paris are the same as those they make to fellow Parisians.

Be that as it may, the centers of Lacanian activity in Paris in 1973 were, first, the Ecole freudienne de Paris, a combined association and institute that Lacan had founded in 1964; second, the Seminar, a weekly or bi-weekly lecture Lacan had been offering since the early fifties and which by 1973 was one of the longest running Parisian fads in memory; third, the University of Paris at Vincennes, where a psychoanalysis department had been spreading the "message" since 1968; and fourth, psychoanalytic and psychotherapeutic practice, Lacan's and that of people influenced by him (by 1973 this was a substantial number, destined to grow significantly throughout the seventies).

Let me begin, somewhat at random, with the Seminar, a center of Parisian intellectual activity. Over the years people like Barthes, Leiris, Derrida, Althusser, Merleau-Ponty, Jakobson, Ricoeur, Sollers, Kristeva, and many others had attended Lacan's lectures. His influence on French intellectual life derived from these lectures more than from his writings—his ideas circulated by word of mouth well before they became enshrined in print. One book that was strongly influenced by the Seminar was Paul Ricoeur's *Freud and Philosophy*, where there is no acknowledgment of Lacan as a formative influence. Lacan found this outrageous and denounced Ricoeur for plagiarizing him. Apparently the weight of the evidence was sufficiently strong for the charges to be accepted by many French intellectuals. Another incident occurred when Gilles Deleuze and Félix Guattari published *Anti-Oedipus*. They intended it as an attack on Lacan and as a challenge to him, and according to Michel Foucault the authors were intensely interested in hearing what Lacan would say about it during his Seminar. However, honor and pride prevented the authors from attending themselves, so they sent Deleuze's wife in their stead for three weeks running. Not one to talk to stand-ins, Lacan kept resolutely silent about the book.

The cultural influence of the Seminar was officially acknowledged in the fall of 1968 at the Ecole normale supérieure where Lacan had been giving the lectures since 1964. The director of that august institution decided that the student uprising of May 1968 had been spawned by Lacan's Seminar and that he would no longer be permitted to give it on the campus at the rue d'Ulm. Lacan responded by saying that the director reminded him of one of those chains you pull when you flush a toilet; this mobilized student outrage and the director found his office occupied by Lacanians, in confirmation of his suspicions about the subversiveness of Lacan. Lacan's relations with the insurgents were never all that clear-cut, however. Once at Vincennes he told a group of revolutionary students that he could not be expected to have an intelligent dialogue with them because they didn't even know what aphasia was. The students were incensed, and one protested on the spot by taking his clothes off. Lacan responded that he had seen better the night before.

The Seminar was an event: at any given time there were

more tape recorders in operation than there were people at the seminars of Lévi-Strauss, Foucault, or Barthes. Lacan spoke to an audience of approximately 800 people squeezed into a room meant for 650. The performance was theatrical: he knew how to deliver a lecture with flair and grace, to address his audience directly, giving you the feeling that he was talking to you personally. The subject matter was always abstract and obscure, but being there to hear it from the master gave people the sense of participating in an important intellectual event that was invariably stimulating.

For the academic year 1972–73 the seminar topic was femininity and the title was "Encore." This seminar spoke to women in a way that few psychoanalytic texts have ever done, and it exerted an important influence on French feminism. Later Lacan would be denounced as a phallocrat, an unrepentant champion of phallic values, but in 1973 he was read and studied with great respect by feminists; he was considered to be one of those who had made an important contribution to the study of femininity.

If no analyst before or since has done as well with the question of femininity, it would be safe to assume that it is not a harmless issue. Philippe Sollers told me that the reason Lacan waited until he was seventy-one to broach the issue was that he knew the kinds of negative aftereffects it would produce. Women would never forgive Lacan for saying that they were not everything and, what was worse, men would never forgive him either. But one must also say that Lacan was a man who loved women, who loved them too well and too much. As I understand the seminar, Lacan was saying that, whatever it is that women want, it is not love. This is not to say that love is unimportant or peripheral in considering femininity; rather that women do not give their love to men who love them, but to men who want them. I think Lacan felt that this conclusion had imposed itself on him and that he also would have preferred leaving these questions to women themselves. For a man to speak truthfully about femininity seems to many people to be a violation of something sacred, an act of theft, of the theft of knowledge. Most people believe that knowledge is firmly grounded only in lived experience; if this were true, then Lacan had nothing to say about femininity or, better, nothing that he could have said would have had a ring of truth. So not only did Lacan violate the sacred mystery of femininity, but he moved to subvert the blind faith people still have in the truthfulness of their "lived experience," in the evidence of their emotional states.

Lacan had said in the early fifties that Freud's discovery was Promethean. The International Psychoanalytic Association had become what it had become because Freud had no confidence in the people to whom he entrusted his discovery. Lacan thought that Freud had set up a bureaucratic caretaker organization for the sole purpose of not letting the fire go out. Lacan believed that Freud did not expect his followers to advance the theory of psychoanalysis; he wanted it guarded until someone else came along to pick up the flame.

Thus Lacan offered what he called a true reading of Freud. In fact, he was embezzling the text from the IPA, taking it from its rightful owners, assuming that there is such a thing as ownership of a text. Lacan's true reading is closer to being a misreading. Despite what he says, it is difficult to criticize the IPA because its members tend to read Freud as a canonical text, repeating it verbatim, without asking too many questions. How can this reading be wrong if it is simply a retranscription of what Freud himself wrote?

It can and it is: anyone who has not misread a text has not read it either. This is a point well made by Harold Bloom. Anyone who has not entered into a dialogue with a text, who has not asked it questions and listened to its answers, not attempted to find within it even better answers, not selected some parts for special emphasis while omitting consideration of others, anyone who has not done this has not read the text. The problem with this kind of reading is that it requires training. The training may come from literary criticism or philosophy, but no one knows instinctively how to read a text and no one learns how to do it by studying natural science.

The original rationale for Lacan's seminar was to teach psychoanalysts how to read Freud. Since most analysts in the early fifties were psychiatrists, this was a necessary endeavor. Lacan did not pay attention to the voice of reason, which should have told him that physicians are not well disposed to such activities. By and large Lacan was successful here. His people learned to read Freud with considerable care and intelligence, and they were a very literate group; much like the early analysts, they were men and women of culture. Even the writings of those French analysts who did not have contact with Lacan show the influence of Lacan's prescription for close study of Freud's work. By 1973 Lacan had passed beyond this stage of his teaching. At the end of the seminar "Encore" he introduced a subject that he felt was the culmination of his work, the *pons asinorum* of his theory.

For quite some time European intellectuals had held the suspicion that something was radically wrong with metaphysical philosophy, with the way we think things and conceptualize experience. But it is one thing to show where philosophy went wrong, and quite another to propose an alternate structure that will set things on a better course. The first enterprise is critical in the largest sense: it involves a reading of texts, an analysis or deconstruction of those texts to reveal a point of contradiction or even a flaw. Here one is reader or explicator. Lacan's efforts to teach people to read Freud were not strictly critical enterprises; they involved learning how to listen selectively rather than how to write criticism. The second enterprise, that of constructing a theory to be read and studied, is where Lacan's research was always heading, even when he was teaching people how to read. He expected that they would ultimately be able to read Lacan.

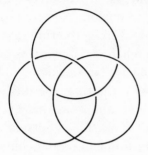

So around 1973 Lacan introduced what one may call the Lacanian thing: the Borromean knot. The last years of the Seminar, which ended in 1980, would be dedicated to the elaboration of the structure of this knot. As always, Lacan proceeded in slow and painstaking fashion. I can't explain here all of the wonderful things you can do with Borromean knots. Suffice it to say that Lacan believed that the Euclidean geometry of planes, lines, solids, and spheres had omitted a crucial element, the ring, which is the most elementary form of a knot. The significance of the ring lies in the fact that if your thought is based on the concept of an enclosed space—a sphere—you use that space to make a primary differentiation between what is inside and what is outside. You may even be led to divide things up into an inner world and an outer reality, even to seek an accommodation of the two.

The faculty Lacan associated with this tendency was consciousness. As Daniel Dennett put it in the introduction to *The Mind's I:* "Our ordinary concept of consciousness seems to be anchored to two separate sets of considerations that can be captured roughly by the phrases 'from the inside' and 'from the outside.'" With only a very few exceptions, psychoanalytic theory is mired in this spherical way of conceptualizing things. People are advised to integrate things or parts of the self; they are advised to express emotions and feelings; to introspect and to extroject. When the psyche holds together in such a world, it does so because the elements of mental life find themselves within the same sack, from which alien and noxious elements have been expelled.

Once the base structure is the ring instead of the sphere, things change. Lacan had said as early as 1952 that any point in the center of a ring can be considered to be either inside or outside the ring. With the ring, the dualism of inside/outside loses its force: you cannot say that a ring contains things within it or that it expels things outside it. For Lacan this posed the following problem: if the containing capacity of the sphere or sack is eliminated, what makes things hold together psychically? His answer was that the elements of mental life are organized according to the structure of the chain or knot. This is not at all the same as what R. D. Laing was talking about in *Knots*. Lacan does not want to untie knots; knotting is not a distinctly negative activity. He wanted to take knots that were tied one way and to tie them another way. There usually is an unknotting before there is a reknotting, but that is a transitory phenomenon. For Lacan a true unknotting represents the psychic disintegration one sees in schizophrenic breakdowns. He did not find this a desirable state.

The Borromean knot is a linkage of three rings in such a way that no two rings intersect. Since the interlocking of any two rings is prohibited, the hole of each of the rings remains inviolate: no other ring can be said to be either inside it or outside it. Since no two rings intersect, but are joined only by the correct placement of the third, the structure of the knot is such that the cutting of any one ring will liberate all of the others. The same principle holds for any number of rings above the number three.

This is not the place to explore all the implications of this topology of knots. Lacan was preoccupied with these questions over the last years of his Seminar. The task he had set himself was nothing less than the subversion of the concept of space that had informed metaphysical philosophy. I include this brief picture of Lacan's theory because this is where he was at when I arrived in Paris. The question of where he was at cannot be answered without taking his theoretical elaborations into account. The theory was the base on which the practice was built, and thus the theory shows where one is at more truly than any empirical gauge.

Still, the more abstract Lacan became, the more he was criticized for working so much on theory. Some thought that while Lacan was fiddling around with knots Paris was going up in smoke. It was said that Lacan was losing touch with the concrete reality of clinical practice. André Green wrote an obituary on Lacan for *Le Monde* in which he said that Lacan could have been a great psychoanalyst but that he squandered his energies trying to build a theory.

The idea of being a great psychoanalyst is a thinly veiled allusion to the idea of being a great physician. The great physician, in our time, does not bother himself with the theory of medicine: he practices, he acts, and he cures people. If a treatment is effective as a curative agent and if it does not pose unacceptable risks, the physician has a duty to prescribe it. The physician does not theorize about the psychological implications of taking a medicine, except insofar as psychology helps or hinders the progress toward cure. The theory of medicine is not something that physicians give very much thought to. As medicine has become increasingly technical and precise, physicians have become increasingly isolated from their patients as speaking subjects. It is not the patients' words that count, but the results of the lab tests. All of this makes medicine more effective, it would seem, and this effectiveness is valid whether or not the physician knows anything about the theory of medicine, and even at times whether or not he knows why the treatment works.

For Lacan, psychoanalytic theory and practice were linked in such a way that a failure of the one involved the eventual degradation of the other. Theory and practice are knotted, and the elimination of either one would send the other off into space. He practiced his theory, and theory building was for him an ongoing enterprise, a kind of interminable analysis. (*I* should note that the requirement that analysts know theory does not require them to be either makers of theory or teachers of theory; these activities are properly supplementary.) The interplay of theory and practice was such that Lacan often said that major points of his theory were taught to him by his analysands. However abstract and abstruse Lacan's theoretical elucubrations were, the people who were listening to them at the Seminar generally found things that spoke to them.

The problem of the interrelation between theory and practice cannot be posed as an either-or proposition. From what I have been saying it sounds like an if-and-only-if proposition. But from the standpoint of the Borromean knot, if theory and practice are rings, then there is no way to connect them in Borromean fashion if we have only these two rings or, better, if we cannot count beyond two. What we want to know is: What is the third ring in this psychoanalytic circus? For Lacan the third ring was the real; in the present context that real can only be the psychoanalyst's existence, which Lacan would have written "ex-sistence." Among the many virtues of the idea of existence, the word itself as Lacan used it, means standing forth, emerging from, with the prefix emphasizing the "outsideness"of the stance. This implies that when we ask about the analyst's existence we are really asking about something that takes place outside of sessions, separate from professional activity. Why else would psychoanalysis have the peculiar requirement that those who wish to be analysts should themselves undergo analysis—why, if not to be assured that these people have something of an ex-sistence? I am not saying for the moment what constitutes this ex-sistence, simply that it ought to be there. Ex-sisting, I hasten to add, is not at all the same as being alive.

If it is desirable that psychoanalysts exist outside of the sessions they conduct, what do they do within those sessions? One answer might be that they insist. Precisely, they insist that nothing real should happen in the session, that the patient should not establish an existence within the space and time of his sessions. This could be taken as another way of stating the fundamental principle of analysis: that the analyst ought to separate his private from his professional life. Analysts are admonished against socializing with their patients, against seeing them outside sessions, and certainly against sexual contact or marriage. They ought also to be warned against making analysis into the totality of their existence. Now some of this has of course been taken to extremes—there are times when socializing is inevitable—but the principle is nonetheless true. All I am saying here is that this is something that all analysts know in one form or another and that I am articulating in a sightly different fashion, stressing the structural relationship between theory, practice, and the analyst's ex-sistence. Nothing I have said would lend credence to the idea that the more normal an analyst is, the better analyst he will be, that being fully analyzed himself—whatever that means—he will be able to act with his intuitions instead of firmly grounded theoretical principles.

Nothing real happens in a psychoanalysis; the real must always remain outside. Perhaps because Lacan was hysterical and histrionic, he saw analysis as akin to theater. Its base and foundation are to be found in a specific theatrical genre, which I will call high comedy. It is rare indeed that an analysand will see things this way; analysands usually have other genres in mind. Anything but comedy, for comedy lacks seriousness and most analysands want above all to be taken seriously. The analyst ought to remember that in Shakespearean comedy several plots go on at the same time at different levels, and also that the resolution of the central plot will resolve all the subplots. The main plot in psychoanalysis is the transference, but this does not mean that it is the only plot.

There has always been a conflict among psychoanalysts over the question of the emphasis to be placed on theory and practice. In the American Psychoanalytic Association, this was resolved by the simple ploy of limiting analytic training to physicians. Lately the American group has been moving in the direction of opening training to clinical psychologists, thus bringing it in line with other institutes. This is all to the better, but the point to be made is that the major Freudian institution in the United States has for most of its existence been an organization of physicians. This fact alone has had serious consequences for the quality of theoretical work.

An organization that emphasizes practice and that excludes from training those people whose background qualifies them to do advanced theoretical work—I am talking essentially of people trained in the humanities—may well become a theoretical wasteland. Bringing a group of physicians together to discuss questions that have for centuries been posed and debated by philosophers might produce some amusing moments, but it is inconceivable that such untrained people will say anything new and original about those questions, unless they are in a constant interaction with people whose preanalytic training is broader and more intellectually oriented.

Things were different at the Ecole freudienne while I was there. Lacan had opened the doors to lay analysts: there were no formal admissions requirements, no degrees that one had to possess to be considered for membership. Meetings and courses at the Ecole were open to anyone who happened by, free of charge. Lacan's own interaction with philosophers and artists during the thirties had broadened the base for psychoanalysis in France, and when Lacan was giving his Seminar at the Ecole normale supérieure during the mid-sixties he managed to attract some of the best young philosophical minds in France to his school.

It was probably the young philosophy students who were responsible for the popularization of Lacan's teaching in the sixties. These same philosophy students were leaders of the uprising of May 1968. If, as Sherry Turkle has suggested in *Psychoanalytic Politics*, the events of that time contributed to Lacan's popularity, then these students should be held responsible, not necessarily for causing the demonstrations but for channeling energy toward Lacan. Lacan himself was thought to be sympathetic to the students in 1968. Nevertheless he did tell the students of Vincennes that they were puppets of the regime and that they were looking for a Master. He added his belief that they would find one. Several years later he said that the one they had found was him.

The year 1973 marked an important date in this history because it marked the return of Lacan's daughter and son-in-law to Paris. In the forefront of the student uprising, Judith and Jacques-Alain Miller had been dismissed from their posts in the Paris university system and had been exiled to teach in a lycée in Besançon.

Miller did not merely return to Paris: he returned to teaching in the department of psychoanalysis at the University of Paris at Vincennes, to participating in meetings at the Ecole, to editing Lacan's seminars for publication, and to editing a new psychoanalytic journal, called *Ornicar?* He also returned at a time when the question of Lacan's heir was becoming more and more pressing, and his appearance on the scene made him look like the successor. That all posed a problem: Miller was not a psychoanalyst and had not even been psychoanalyzed. Later he rectified these lapses, but at the time he represented a challenge and a threat to the established medical professionals, most of whom had long been loyal to Lacan. People feared that Lacan would leave psychoanalysis in the hands of a nonanalyst, and one who was openly contemptuous of the older, wiser, more experienced practitioners. In 1973 Miller was around thirty years old: the very image of the upstart who was using his family position to advance his career. What was perceived as Miller's position can be caricatured in a statement attributed to him but that, to my knowledge, he never made: How can the older analysts think of themselves as Lacanians when they don't even know Descartes or Hegel?

Miller was not alone: not only did he have Lacan's support, but quite a few of Miller's former classmates at the Ecole normale and many of his students from Vincennes were in training at the Ecole. By 1974 about half the analysts of the Ecole were nonphysicians and, at the time of the dissolution (1980), the figure had risen to three quarters. There was then considerable sympathy for Miller among the Young Turks of the Ecole, and no lack of antipathy from older analysts who were not getting much respect for the work they had put it. Another point that ought to be emphasized is that in debates at congresses and meetings the younger people generally had the upper hand. They were masters of complex theoretical elaboration, and in a head-to-head rhetorical battle with a psychiatrist there was no contest.

This situation did not come about only because Lacan respected philosophers, linguists, mathematicians, and the like, or because he was a champion of lay analysis. It occurred because, when push came to vote within the analytic institutes in Paris, Lacan could not count on the analysts to support him, could not count on the medical analysts to take his side, no matter what their debt or obligation to him.

Look at the path Lacan followed to get to the Ecole normale in 1964. In 1963 the International Psychoanalytic Association issued an ultimatum to the association that Lacan led: Lacan would have to give up doing training analysis and teaching in the institute if the group wished to be affiliated with the International. He would have to terminate all of the training analyses he was doing. This would have had more than symbolic consequences for a man who had large numbers of people in training with him.

The association put the question to a vote: Lacan's head or affiliation with the IPA. And the group voted for the IPA, against Lacan. The next day Lacan announced that he would no longer give his Seminar at the Hospital Center of Ste. Anne, and the Seminar that year, announced to be "The Name of the Father," would never be given at all. Eventually Lacan found his way to the Ecole normale through the intervention of Lévi-Strauss, Merleau-Ponty, and Althusser.

If Lacan's demands for loyalty became excessive at a later date, I think it is clear that in this case they were not. Many of those who voted that Lacan was incompetent as a training analyst had done their training with him; and they considered themselves to be well trained. And most of those who voted that Lacan should not teach psychoanalysis had attended his Seminar faithfully for years and had learned most of what they knew of analysis from him. Why then did they vote as they did? Was the allure of international respectability so important to them? Did they feel that they needed to be aligned with an organization founded by Freud himself? Maybe so, but Lacan also had a very lucrative practice, composed largely of people in training, and the thought of dividing up that practice no doubt had some influence on the vote.

The Miller story heated up significantly in 1974. The place of the confrontation was the University of Paris at Vincennes. This university rose out of the ashes of the 1968 uprising, created to placate the more radical students. One of the novelties of Vincennes was the existence of a department of psychoanalysis headed by Serge Leclaire. Leclaire is an important character in this drama because he was generally considered to be Lacan's heir-apparent at the time. By 1974 the program in psychoanalysis had failed to live up to Lacan's expectations. As I understood it, the analysts who were brought into this alien environment did not know how to teach. In doubt, they did what they always did; they kept silent. The silence of the analyst-instructor often lasted for many minutes and had the inestimable advantage of signifying to the assembled auditors that the instructor was a real psychoanalyst. The effect was to transform classes into encounter groups: what counted was the experience and not the instruction. In other classes instructors did talk, though what they talked about was not psychoanalysis but their own theories of philosophy. Some placed a great premium on having original theories.

It is clear that someone like Jacques-Alain Miller, a professional educator, could not look too kindly on this peculiar perversion of the educational process. The idea of holding classes as therapy groups also raises a moral issue: people come to a university to be educated; not to be analysed. To submit them to an analytic treatment without their having requested it is highly dubious ethically.

In the fall of 1974 Lacan decided that enough was enough at Vincennes, and he announced that he was going to take over the psychoanalysis department. This was typical of Lacan, especially since officially he had nothing to do with Vincennes, he was not on the staff, and he had no legal right to say anything about what was going on in the department. His justification was that all of the nonsense taking place there was happening in his name and with his implicit approval. So he said that explicitly he did not approve and that he wanted to reorganize the department, with himself as scientific director and with Miller, Charles Melman, and Jean Clavreul as the resident ruling committee. Many saw this act as a premonition of things to come in the Ecole freudienne.

How did Lacan get away with this? In the first place, there was no one around who was about to say no to the great man. The same consideration came to the forefront a year later when the new department decided it was going to give doctorates in psychoanalysis. The minister of education in France was reported to have said that he could not say no to a proposal signed by Lacan without making himself look like a fool around the globe. The same thing happened when the department wanted to give out diplomas in clinical psychoanalysis. As Lacan put it, the reason for his action was to prevent the psychologists from taking over the field by default.

Even as scientific director Lacan had nothing to say about the tenured and nontenured faculty. Thus his efforts at reform were directed at the *chargé de cours* slot. People in this position taught one course per semester and were paid something like $40 per week. Lacan declared that courses in the department would have to offer serious instruction in the theory of psychoanalysis and that anyone who wanted to profess should submit a course summary of five pages detailing what he intended to teach. This was open to anyone, in principle.

When the names of those chosen to teach were posted, there was an outcry, not so much against those chosen—I was among them—but for those who had been excluded. One intellectual luminary who was not chosen was Luce Irigaray, whose theoretical work had increasingly become estranged from Lacan's positions. This was generally taken to be the reason for her exclusion, and it raised protest to the effect that Lacan was interested only in promoting dogma.

The French are not generally very big on eclecticism; not all points of view have to be aired, they feel. Lacan thought that there were right and wrong ways of presenting psychoanalytic theory—by which he meant his theory—and that in a department he headed he should have something to say about how theory was taught. So there were exclusions and this, along with the entire affair, was such an affront to the university system that people like Gilles Deleuze and Jean-François Lyotard tried to mount a campaign against Lacan—which ultimately failed.

The mid-seventies were great years for the psychoanalysis department at Vincennes. I myself taught there from 1974 through 1977. What was impressive was that, as soon as the department became known for offering serious courses, students flocked in. The introductory-level courses were attended consistently by well over one hundred people. The program in clinical psychoanalysis was always oversubscribed, and the review *Ornicar?* had reached a circulation surpassing that of the well-known *Tel Quel.* Certainly the fact that Lacan's seminars came to be published in *Ornicar?* helped.

In the winter of 1980–81 things changed dramatically. The place of confrontation was the program in clinical psychoanalysis. This program was comprised of case presentations, seminars, discussion groups, and practical work in selected Paris hospitals. The directors of the program had forged links with several hospitals that received candidates in the program to teach them about practice firsthand. The program was in the hands of psychiatrists who were also Lacanian psychoanalysts.

The rest of the department was thought to be under the control of Jacques-Alain Miller. It was thought that Miller was using the department to establish a power base for himself, through his publications, programs, and lecture series, and that from this base he would move on to take control of the new Cause freudienne, created from the Ecole Lacan had dissolved the year before. Also it was alleged that since Miller was a professor he was going to make the Cause into a universitylike enterprise, thus diminishing the influence of the psychiatrist-analysts. The psychiatrists were led by Charles Melman, one of Lacan's most devoted students, and also Miller's analyst.

It all came down to a conflict between Miller and Melman. First Melman denounced the high-handed tactics he thought Miller used to compose the statutes of the Cause; second he denounced the handling of the disposition of property of the old school. Now the psychiatrists who had been a part of the program in clinical psychoanalysis resigned en masse, declaring that students from the program would no longer be welcome on their services. This was the beginning of a veritable war of words in which Miller was attacked with some of the most vituperative prose it has ever been my misfortune to read. This is not to say that Miller is or was angelic; only that, no matter what he did, the cause of psychoanalysis could never have been served by the torrents of hatred that flowed from the pens of Parisian analysts. The fact that Miller's analyst was leading the opposition gave a particularly sordid quality to the debate.

Where was Lacan through all of this? He remained silent. On occasion Lacan would issue a statement of support for Miller, but this only served to fuel the rage of those who were opposed to Miller. They accused him of sequestering Lacan, of forcing him to sign statements he had not written, of manipulating Lacan like a puppet to promote his own ambitions. I considered these charges to be implausible to an extreme. Those who had originally been against the ascendance of Miller because he was not analyzed and did not practice analysis were even more horrified when it was disclosed that he had been doing an analysis and that he was beginning to receive patients in analysis. This seemed to suggest that Jacques-Alain Miller was about to name himself supreme psychoanalytic autocrat, that he wanted to have everything, and that psychiatrists would no longer be masters of their own house. On the other side, Miller did alienate a very large number of Lacan's most faithful disciples in an extremely brief period of time, so it would be difficult to say that he handled the situation faultlessly.

Whatever side one takes, it is clear that the disintegration of the world of Lacanian psychoanalysis was not a pretty spectacle. It created some horrendous press for psychoanalysis and discouraged people from seeking analytic treatment. The general public is no doubt wrong in expecting analysts to be models of behavior—this is nothing more than a bourgeois ideal. And yet a large number of Parisian analysts did manage to make fools of themselves in the conflicts of 1979–1981, in ways beyond ex-sistence and ex-centricity. No one could reproach analysts for having passions, but passions by definition are suffered, not acted upon, certainly not spewed forth as if the goal of analysis were to be led around by one's passions and to exhibit them proudly in public. Too many people did so, and in the end it was the cause of psychoanalysis that suffered the most.

In the midst of the polemics one thing is observable: Lacan ultimately lost the support of just about all of the psychiatrists he trained. The magnitude of this phenomenon makes it impossible to say that these people were ignoble, ungrateful, or dishonorable. There is only so much blame we can allot here before we are obliged to ask whether there was not something in Lacan himself that made this inevitable. I have already spoken of Lacan's hubris, of the autocratic control he seemed to exert over his students and disciples, of the passion for revenge that may well have arisen from this. But it is not useful to pin this on the back of one man. The splits and schisms in French psychoanalysis were not isolated phenomena; they happened in similar form in most psychoanalytic societies, from Vienna to Berlin to New York, and they happened whether or not Lacan was the issue.

Perhaps the solitary nature of analytic practice makes it impossible for analysts to form groups. Perhaps the kind of social relation that pertains in analysis is so satisfying that no other kind of social relation can hold much interest for analysts. These were some of the arguments advanced in Paris. And yet it may very well be that there is an intrinsic or basic flaw in psychoanalysis itself, in Freudian psychoanalysis. Many people have suspected such a thing, but they have tended to want to discard Freud just because they have discovered where he went astray. Perhaps the story I have just told will give us a clue: it appears that the flaw in psycho-analysis derives from its base in medicine, from the idea that it ought to be a curative enterprise.

What is wrong with psychoanalysis is that it has as a goal, and as a reason for being, the medical model of treatment and cure. The ideals of mental health and mental hygiene have nothing to do with existence, even though it is true that someone who is symptom-ridden, who suffers from a neuro-sis, will not have attained much of an existence. The point I am making here is that the converse is not true: being symp-tom-free, being healthy, is not the same as existing.

3

PSYCHOANALYSIS WAS DISCOVERED BY A VIENNESE NEU-
rologist named Freud. It was dubbed the talking cure by the
first analytic patient, Bertha Pappenheim, or Anna O. She
was not Freud's patient; her physician was Josef Breuer who
consulted with his colleague Freud on the case. Freud was
not the first to undertake an analytic treatment, but rather
the first to offer analytic supervision.

Psychoanalysis developed as an attempt to treat untreat-
able patients. Its goal was cure, and its practitioners have by
and large been physicians. It has even spawned a subspeci-
ality called psychotherapy, which relates to analysis roughly
in the same way that physiotherapy relates to medical treatment. There is no basic contradiction between psychiatry
and psychology as far as a goal is concerned. And so long as
psychoanalysis thinks that it too holds as its goal the attain-
ment of cure, so long as it judges treatment by results, it too
will find fulfillment within the medical community.

Freud had the sense that what he was proposing was very
radical indeed. He did not expect his fellow medical practitioners to greet his discovery with the proverbial open arms.
They did not. There has always been a tension created by

the efforts of analysts to get themselves recognized as part of the medical community and by the physicians' attitude of suspicion toward analysis. After all, doctors have enough trouble thinking of psychiatry as medicine. Despite the fact that analysts love to make analogies between their practice and surgery, no surgeon will ever accept the comparison with anything other than haughty condescension. You don't have to be an analyst to recognize the implications of begging for acceptance by a group that simply does not want you.

And so Lacan said that psychoanalysis did not have as its goal curing patients, and that if people in analysis did get better it was a welcome side effect. The statement caused considerable commotion in France. If analysis does not want to cure, then it cannot be classed as a medical subspecialty: it is trying to do something that is alien to medicine. Thus the physicians, the real ones, are right to be suspicious of analysis. But then, you may ask, where are we to classify analysis? Some say it is educational, others that it is a religious experience. Lacan said that it was none of the above, that it was psychoanalysis and that it was different.

Was he saying something that people didn't know? Probably not. He was saying something that no one wanted to admit because the social acceptance of analysis was based, in the minds of many, on the idea that it could provide cures. People who go to analysts are suffering and they seek to have that suffering alleviated, just as when they go to see a doctor. If analysis does not hold out the promise of cure, then people won't go into analysis. So goes the thought of many people in the profession, and understandably. The only problem is that if it were simply a question of reducing suffering, why not take a pill? The little pill is more effective in many cases, it works quicker, and it costs much less. Thus it happens that in the marketplace of the mental health professions there are far more people who are taking pills, or who are engaged in short-term therapeutic procedures, than there are in analysis. By calling itself a branch of medicine, psychoanalysis has put itself in a position where it cannot compete, except perhaps with grandiose promises of supercures. Unfortunately, it has never been able to demonstrate the validity of any of the more grandiose promises.

I will thus ask a question that is probably the only one in which the idea of cure can properly be related to psychoanalysis: Can psychoanalysis be cured of medicine, of the belief that it is part of the healing professions? Can physicians who become analysts ever part with the idea that their analytic practice is grounded in their medical expertise?

If the experience of Lacan is any indication, the answer must be a guarded no. He tried to introduce a break between psychoanalysis and medicine. Not that he ever denied being a psychiatrist, but his theorization has nothing whatever to do with medicine or even with natural science. We can say that he was preceded by Freud who said in *The Question of Lay Analysis* that the study of medicine will give no advantage in reading psychoanalytic texts. And he was followed by Jacob Arlow, a respected American analyst, who said that medical training is a handicap for the study of analysis.

Lacan was on this track, and he went farther than anyone else. Yet he still failed; almost all of his psychiatry students left him in the end. Is this simply proof of the impossibility of detaching analysis from medicine? And if the task is impossible, perhaps we should drop it and content ourselves with redefining the idea of cure. Otherwise we might want to ponder the idea that the psychiatrists trained by Lacan were themselves not strong enough to renounce medicine and all that it affords in rewards and glory. This would be an interesting argument to make; the problem is that in France the position of senior analyst provided plenty of rewards and glory. In the United States, where the American Psychoanalytic Association has tried to institutionalize the medical roots of analysis, psychiatrists who choose analysis do make very real sacrifices: if they want money and fame they will have done better to stick with psychiatry. In part this disparity has to do with the differing social status of the physician in different countries; it also relates to the fact that in France medicine is socialized whereas analysis is not. One could probably make the argument that the factors contributing to the tremendous interest in psychoanalysis in France were, first, the socialization of medicine with the government's control over fees; second, the unemployment rates for philosophy students who sought an academic career; third, the fact that psychoanalysis in France was traditionally a cash business—the implications of this fact do not need elaboration. In any case, the comparison between France and America in terms of the place of medicine in analysis is interesting, even paradoxical, but it still leaves open the question of whether analysis can be cured of medicine.

And I would like to approach the question theoretically. To introduce it I will quote some remarks Robert Jay Lifton made to me concerning Lacan's death. Lifton, an authority on holocausts and other castastrophic human events, is something of an intellectual loner for his espousal of the importance of something that analysts, among others, have never wanted to look at very closely: death and its symbolization. I think that the crux of the matter of the separation of medicine and psychoanalysis has to do with the symbolization of death. After all, the physicians of the American Psychoanalytic Association, the most Freudian group in this country, have never had any use for Freud's concept of the death drive.

Lifton met Lacan at Yale in 1975 and asked him about the symbolization of death. He proposed this as an alternative to the classical psychoanalytic symbolization that centers on sex and sexual relations. Why couldn't there be another system of symbolization besides the one focused on male and female principles? That other symbolization would be of continuity and discontinuity or better, he added, continuity and death. Lacan responded: "I am a Liftonian." Of course, everyone thought this to be a facetious remark, a kind of mock praise. And yet it was not characteristic of Lacan to give compliments, and besides he knew better than most that there is always truth in wit.

What Lacan said next makes this clear. He stated that he was a Freudian and that the Freudian approach emphasized sex, adding that he was probably too old to change. He thought that Lifton's approach might be just as valid as his own, since there was more than one path that research could follow. Perhaps they would end up at the same place. It was certainly true that Lacan tended to urge people to follow the lines opened by their own work; he did not demand that everyone work on what he was working on, or even that they work in exactly the same way theoretically.

This brief exchange is significant for what followed in Paris. If the events of the last few years tell us anything, they demonstrate that psychoanalysts have a difficult time with death, that the symbolization of death was not functional in the Ecole freudienne, at least as far as the death of Lacan was concerned, and that Lacan's death was something that the institution could not handle. This is intriguing because Lacan did not shrink before theorization about death. He had a theory about the desire for death, and he was one of the few post-Freudian analysts who did not write off the death drive.

The third section of Lacan's "Function and Field" is a prime example, but the unpublished seminar "The Ethics of Psychoanalysis" (1959–60) is also relevant. There he emphasized the importance of the tragedy of *Antigone* and especially of the *ate*, the essential calamity that inhabits the play. Let me note that *Antigone* is not a play about Oedipal rivalry, but rather about the relationship between the living and the dead. But Lacan was far more in his element when he spoke of love and desire and sexuality. Perhaps it is significant that in his later seminars Lacan replaced the theme of death with a theme that is synonymous, that of the sexual satisfaction of *jouissance*. This topic was certainly more congenial to Lacan's audience: it was sexier to talk about orgasms than to ponder the fate of the dead. Yet we know that sexual satisfaction has often been described by poets as signifying death.

Lacan's choice of the Hegelian dialectic of master and slave as the model for the relations of consciousness and the world, for the imaginary order, places death, the absolute master, to the side; no one dies in the Hegelian myth. In the struggle for prestige one of the two combatants gives up before the moment of truth, and he thereby becomes the slave. His defeat is a signal of fear or apprehension before death, fear that Lacan later said was insignificant in comparison to the apprehension about living too long.

Now there is a murder in the Oedipal myth as it is articulated by Freud. And yet, since Freud tends to state the myth in terms of the intention to murder rather than of the murder itself, there is here a similar putting of death to the side. This is perhaps most evident in the idea that the living father, threatened by his sons, will want to castrate them.

The one place where Freud took the role of the dead into account fully was in writing about the primal horde. There he said that, once the first father was murdered, he became identified with the Law and this Law was far more ferocious and inhibiting than the real father had been. Lacan was in fact well aware of the psychoanalytic failure to symbolize death. His critique of the Freudian Oedipus complex states that the privilege accorded to the act of murder was actually a wish to revive and resuscitate the father, who was father, who occupied the paternal function fully, only insofar as he was dead. As Lacan once said, Freud so loved his father that he revived him to give him all women.

Lacan thus advanced the theory on this question, but probably did not take it far enough. What if, instead of the Hegelian myth of master and slave, Lacan had begun with the story of Cain and Abel. Instead of the imperatives of the master, he would have had to deal with the phenomena of malediction and sacrifice. When Lacan considered the text of Genesis in his ill-fated seminar on the name of the father, the passage he chose was that of the sacrifice of Isaac by Abraham, a story of salvation, of saving someone from the grasp of death.

Neither Lacan nor Freud was ignorant of the problem posed by the dead. What I am saying is that events in Paris show that Lacan did not take things far enough. To do so he would have run up against the medical juggernaut with its passion for life, for saving life, for prolonging life, for beating death. The great advantage then to making symbolism sexual is that it favors the production of life, and even the advancement of the quality of life. But what if the rivalry between father and son, between brother and brother, is not sexual, is not for a sexual object, but is in terms of the worthiness of offerings to the dead, as it is in the story of Cain and Abel? These questions have also been posed by René Girard.

The relationship between medicine and death is not too difficult to define: the function of medical practice is to repress death, thus to favor life—and those things that make life worth living. By and large doctors concern themselves with the living: the dead are the business of undertakers and religious authorities. Society feels a special horror when a physician is charged with causing a death; nowadays this is translated into the turmoil of malpractice litigation.

Basically there are two social institutions that are concerned with the symbolization of death and dying—Freud discusses them in *Group Psychology and the Analysis of the Ego*—the church and the army. Is it not symptomatic that most psychoanalysts are opposed to the existence of both groups, that in some sense they have felt with Freud that the existence of psychoanalysis should make both groups unnecessary. You might think that this is a blind spot, but the location of this blind spot is not insignificant. Most analysts and therapists believe that anyone who kills under whatever circumstances is unhealthy and also that anyone who follows a religion is neurotic. To distinguish the church from the army, we say that the church is concerned with symbolizing the negotiations that must take place between the living and the dead, while the army is concerned with symbolizing, to say nothing of causing, the passage between life and death. The latter poses the most problems, but clearly people are more comfortable about dying within a structured event than about dying naturally; in addition, a death that is part of a social institution symbolizing the passage between life and death is superior to a death that is accidental, asocial, not in the line of socially determined duty and role. This is not too easy to follow, but certainly the idea that we are somehow going to rid the world of war must count as an illusion, not only because people are unremittingly hostile to each other but because wars have a social and symbolizing function that is essential to the coherence of the group.

Psychoanalysis has always been thought of as a therapeutic enterprise, justified by the results it obtains. Even if we admit with Lacan that the goal of analysis is not cure, what then are we to do with the fact that analysis does at times produce clear and palpable benefits for patients? And if it does, why shouldn't the analyst bask in the glow of thinking that he himself is the curative agent? Why shouldn't the analyst think of himself as having mastered and defeated a neurosis? We can understand the considerable narcissistic appeal of such positions. They are a reaction to the argument offered against analysis that its results can be obtained normally through the process of growth or through time. It is difficult if not impossible for analysis to answer such objections, since control experiments are obviously impossible to set up in a scientifically acceptable fashion.

Besides, what are the alternatives? If the analyst is not the agent of cure, then what is? Perhaps the analyst is one who permits a cure to take place because he himself is uninterested in such things. Perhaps the analyst's expectation about cure is a fundamental obstacle on the path to any therapeutic result. Certainly this is one of the points of Lacan's remarks about cure and analysis. This is true as far as it goes, but Lacan's point is more profound. What he was saying was that the direction of analysis ought to lead toward a verbalization of the unconscious. This much analysis generally knows how to do. The question is what this does to the individual who thus learns to verbalize his unconscious. And here we are on more uncertain ground. The process may produce a disappearance of symptoms; it may produce an amelioration in the subject's general attitude toward himself and toward others; it may even make him into a more mature individual, a better person. But there is no guarantee that this will happen. Perhaps our concept of psychic cure is skewed, not because we don't know what a psychic cure is but because the conceptualization of such a thing is unwarranted. It may be that there is no such thing as cure when we are talking about the psyche. The concept of cure in psychoanalysis may go back to a belief that psyche must follow soma, that we can have the same degree of certainty in the one as we think we obtain with the other. Psychoanalysis ought to get out of the business of thinking about how people live their lives, about how they behave. What this means, perhaps unexpectedly, is that analysis has as its major task the repairing of the relationships people have, not with other people, but with the dead.

How did psychoanalysis get into the life business? Freud's first patients were hysterical young women, suffering from problems that prevented them from having normal sexual relations, from loving and desiring men, from settling down into good marriages, from bringing up healthy children. There is something properly insufferable for the physician in the picture of a being who is the very image of fecundity, of the promise of new life, renouncing that for the dubious satisfactions of neurosis. It was what physicians call a life-threatening situation, even species-threatening.

It is one thing to say that hysterical women are suffering from sexual repression, and certainly Freud was very courageous to talk about sexual matters openly with a patient named Dora, as he himself asserts. But it must also be noted that such patients are extremely curious about sexual matters—as the relationship between Dora and Frau K. shows strikingly—and that what matters to them most in life is love. Perhaps it is rare that such a patient will think of sexuality in quite so graphic and detached a way as Freud did, but to say that these matters are not a major preoccupation of women suffering from hysteria is dishonest. After all, it is with hysterical patients that we find the most clearly sexual allegories, the most unmistakable examples of sexual symbolism.

The promotion of sexuality as the privileged content of symbolization has its roots in the fact that analysis was taught to Freud by hysterics. And the discourse of hysteria was said by Lacan to be the closest to the discourse of analysis. The problem is how to get from the one to the other: Does this take place when the allegories of the hysteric are translated into sexual terms and the patient is thus liberated for life and love, for sex and begetting? Not quite. And here one can object not only because such an idea slides the analytic discourse into the hysterical discourse, but also because it represents a failure on the part of the analyst to listen to what his patient is telling him. If the hysteric has renounced life for something else, then we ought to be more curious about what that something else is. It does not take a very careful reading of the case of Anna O. to recognize that the patient is fixated on the scene of her vigil for her dying father. It would appear that the dead have far more appeal to the hysteric than anything about the living has and that hysteria is a failed attempt to stay in touch with the dead. If the analyst promotes the values of life to the hysteric, he is doing nothing more than feeding her repression. The hysteric wants to keep the dead alive, to give them life.

The problem that has to be treated is the relationship with the dead: the hysteric ought to come to mediate that relationship with something other than a conversion symptom. If psychoanalysis remains stuck in sexual symbolism, this is because analysts are by and large faithful lovers, ever faithful to the women who taught them their practice. The question of whether Freud was faithful to his wife is an issue whose importance is primarily theoretical—because the history of psychoanalysis has been marked by the fact that Freud did remain faithful to his first patients. And when I mentioned that some people may have been scandalized by Lacan's womanizing, I don't think that the truth of the matter lies in the details of Lacan's life. It would appear that Lacan's crime was to have been unfaithful to hysteria, to have tried to move the psychoanalytic enterprise in a different direction; for this he was treated to an outpouring of pure and unalloyed hysteria on the part of the people he had trained. On this score Lacan, by his own admission, did not succeed.

In part the question of the symbolization of death was neglected by Lacan because it was relegated to the world of obsessional neurosis. As Serge Leclaire states in his article, "Jerome, or Death in the Life of the Obsessional" (in my *Returning to Freud*), the question for the obsessional is: Am I alive or dead? The hysteric's question is: Am I a man or a woman? If, as Lacan stated, the effect of psychoanalysis is to "hysterize" patients in the transference, then any emphasis on issues that are of particular concern to obsessionals would function as an obstacle to the treatment. Thus Lacan rejected obsessional neurosis as a model for treatment and rejected the concomitant ritualization of the analytic setting, the efforts to strengthen the fortresslike structure of the ego, and the emphasis on the intrapsychic. Lacan promoted the hysterical intersubjectivity, tampered with the time of the analytic session, and considered the ego to be the enemy.

Deconsidering the question of death and the dead does not make it go away. Saying that obsessional neurotics are particularly fascinated with death does not make the question trivial or banal. Thus Lacan was faced with the task of constructing a theory to account for the exchange between the living and the dead, the commerce between the subject and what he called Otherness.

Lacan did not consider psychoanalysis to be an Oedipal enterprise. His goal for treatment was not to create a bunch of Hamlets brooding over their repressed Oedipal longings. For Lacan, Hamlet was the very model of the structure of obsessional neurosis. Certainly Lacan did not discard the Oedipus complex, but he did attempt to take it one step further. His work on *Antigone* is a prime candidate for the honor of expressing clearly man's relation to and debt to the dead. But the basic reformulation involves replacing patricide and incest, taken as objects of consciousness, by theft as a symbolic act.

So Lacan, being perhaps more subtle than was necessary, began his "Function and Field" with the statement that the Freudian discovery of the unconscious was a Promethean discovery and that every analyst in his office repeats that Promethean act. Lacan was somewhat less subtle in choosing as the first essay in the French edition of his *Ecrits* a seminar on Poe's "The Purloined Letter." Some people have suggested that Lacan chose this as a slap at France's resident psychoanalytic expert on Poe, Marie Bonaparte, but the important point is that this story concerns an act of theft.

Relations between the living and the dead never take place in an atmosphere of communication leading to interpersonal and mutual understanding. In place of this humanistic model for therapy, Lacan proposed one based on the elements of theft and sacrifice. Prometheus is the most striking example of this for his stealing of fire from the gods or the immortals. And he does this through the exercise of cunning, of his wits. The gods, however, must have some recompense, for man has through an act placed himself in debt to them. Thus man offers sacrifices that the dead may either accept or reject. Sometimes when a sacrifice is unacceptable, when the dead do not receive their due, they harass and torment and obsess the living. This much we may call ethnological fact.

Does the possession of fire, of speech or the purloined letter, make human beings feel that they are alive? How can one revel in the sense of being alive when that sense is established by the possession of something that is the property of beings who are not alive? (The gods, being immortal, cannot have the same kind of life we revel in when we feel alive.) In his seminar on "The Purloined Letter" Lacan stated that anyone, in this case the unscrupulous minister, who retains a signifier that belongs to someone else will come to be identified with the person who is the rightful possessor of the signifier, here the queen. Possessing fire, then, man felt himself to be a god. Remember that Freud states in his paper "The Acquisition and Control of Fire" that man stole fire when he renounced his urge to extinguish it with urine. Through this renunciation of a "natural" function man accedes to desire. The biological organ, the penis, thereby becomes the signifying phallus.

Thus man did not feel more alive, but he did gain a sense of existing. Philosophers have given more attention to the question of whether God exists than they have to the question of whether God is alive. To wonder whether God is alive or dead is properly an obsessional enterprise. To declare that God is dead is also to state that he once was alive, thus that we are alive if we are strong enough to think that God is dead. If we are merely alive, then we are not identifying with the position of the gods, but rather denying our debt for our theft. We are attempting to circumvent what

Lacan called the Law, which posits that our debt to the gods is not payable in full under any circumstances, not even when we want to pay with our lives.

There are identifications and there are identifications. Some people identify themselves as dead, as the residue or waste product of life. These ambulating cadavers are not in the place where man, having stolen fire, felt himself to be a god. Being dead is not the same as being a corpse. Corpses are only the imaginary representation of death and thus not the entire story. The symbolic representation of death is silence, and the real representation is our gods.

The identification in question concerns the marking of a part of the body, not in the sense that it becomes dead tissue, but rather in the sense that it no longer functions according to the laws of biology. One such part is the phallus, long the subject of considerable mystery, precisely because its workings seem to be different from the workings of other parts of the body. The phallus appears to be marching to its own tune, at times in discord with the will or intentions of the subject; it obeys, one might say, the Other; it functions as a part of speech, as a signifier.

For Prometheus there was a sacrifice of a part of his body, symbolized in the devouring of his liver by a vulture or eagle. But the liver is not a phallic appendage; it has long been considered the locale of the passions. The refusal to make an offering leads to an almost endless cycle of suffering. The signifier of the desire of Zeus, the Other, as far as this punishment is concerned, is the bird.

Obviously Prometheus is alive because otherwise his liver could not regenerate. His existence does not derive from this regeneration but from his sacrifice, through which he comes to desire. This reading, however strange it may seem, states that once Prometheus stole fire, he found himself in a state I will call desiring. This being an unfamiliar state, as unfamiliar as not having a liver, his tendency is to deny his lack, to assert that he is alive and whole, thus permitting his liver to regenerate. The assertion of his being alive is evidence of moral cowardice, of guilt, in that it shows a failure to act with the thing he has stolen. If Prometheus were alive and whole he would be saying that in effect nothing has happened; that gesture is an undoing of what he had done. If Prometheus were permitted to deny his act, he would be destroying the dialectic he has opened between man and the gods, a dialectic in which there is no synthesis, no reconciliation, no redemption.

All told, the dead are not easy to live with. Writing the myth of the primal horde, Freud showed that while the first father prohibited by his presence his sons' access to women, once that father was dead he became the Law that continued the prohibition and obliged the sons to create a structure of marriage in order to avoid perpetual conflict. However difficult the first father was to deal with, once dead he was impossible: unremitting and inexorable.

I am not the first to say that Lacan acted like a tyrannical first father. Disregard the fact that Lacan himself always said that Freud had discovered psychoanalysis—there was in Paris such a cult around Lacan as Master, as the One with all the women, with all the glory, that it was impossible not to identify him with this mythic position. He was not an easy man to get along with; some felt that there was no way of getting along with him at all. Lacan did not teach people how to get along with other people, interpersonally, but rather how to negotiate and to enter into commerce with the dead.

Now this was difficult to understand while Lacan was alive because many people hoped that the man would one day show us his humanity, become one of us, be capable of engaging in small talk as we all do. It was this belief in the life of the Master that was the basis for the psychoanalytic group that formed around Lacan. People were linked together as much by their love for the man as by their adherence to a practice and principles. The events leading up to

Lacan's death show this in stark clarity. Despite what some people have suggestetd, Lacan was never entirely comfortable with the cult of personality, with the glory that attended him. And he tried to transform the structure of the group in the way that one might attempt to move the discourse of hysteria into the discourse of analysis.

To effect this change Lacan introduced into the life of the psychoanalytic group a rite of passage he called *the pass*. It was intended to symbolize the passing of the analysand to the state of the analyst or, for those who were not in training, the passage effected at the termination of a psychoanalysis.

It was with the pass that Lacan suffered his most conspicuous failure. Whatever was involved in the pass, the analytic group was not ready for it. Or else Lacan had miscalculated; he introduced it at the wrong time and with the wrong people. This does not make it any less instructive as an attempt to symbolize death and to realize a commerce with the dead. What Lacan knew and what he wanted to enact was the impossibility of realizing a commerce between the living and the dead in sexual terms. Even more redoubtable was his dictum that commerce between the living and the living dead did not take place in these terms either.

4

IF THERE WERE A TITLE TO THIS CHAPTER, IT COULD BE "Pass or Impasse." And not for reasons of linguistic self-indulgence. There happen to be a wonderful group of expressions that have to do with passing: passing away, passing on, passing through, passing over, to say nothing of passport, password, or making a pass. Some universities have the grading system called pass/fail.

In the Ecole freudienne anyone at any time could decide to do the pass or, as they said in French, *passer la passe.* If you succeeded you were elevated to the rank of *analyste de l'école* (A.E.), which was the highest rank in the school, reserved for those who not only practiced analysis but devoted a considerable part of their energies to teaching and advancing the theory. The rank was roughly equivalent to that of teaching analyst. It did not imply any special privileges as far as training was concerned, since Lacan saw all analysts as competent to conduct training analysis. In principle, the rank of A.E. was not supposed to denote a hierarchical distinction. In practice, those who were accepted in the pass were considered of higher rank than those who had either failed or not tried.

Analysands decided of their own free will to undertake the pass. There was another category of analysts, the *analyste membre de l'école* (A.M.E.), whose members were chosen by committee with the recommendation of the training analyst and supervisor. No demand on the part of the candidate was necessary to be voted A.M.E. This rank signified that the person in question had demonstrated a minimum degree of competence in the private practice of psychoanalysis. Perhaps because of this idea of minimum competence, the A.M.E. title was considered less prestigious than the A.E. At the same time, it generally took longer to become an A.M.E. because one could at any time decide to do the pass. The proper moment was at the point of terminating one's training analysis. Some people who were A.M.E. decided to do the pass, and some of those who did the pass were not A.M.E.

If the pass is to be of interest to us, it must concern more than the professional elevation of the members of the analytic group. If it were simply a more democratic way for people to rise to the top of their profession, little would have been made of it. People would have embraced it enthusiastically. In fact, the institution of the pass caused more conflict and violence than anything except Lacan's invention of the short session.

One could say that psychoanalysis itself was in question in the pass—in question not because its practice was tied into a sexual symbolism, but rather because it posed the question of how that symbolism yielded to a symbolization of death. And it did not yield without some attendant reticence on the part of analysts, a reticence that blossomed almost from the beginning into outright opposition. The fact is that Freud's theories of sexual symbolism had found a following: people liked them, found them challenging and congenial at the same time, and even discovered ways to make use of them commercially. However much these ideas had been repugnant to Victorian Vienna, they were readily accepted in mid-century America and France. Analysts were even heard to say that their patients knew the sexual meaning of their symptoms better than the analysts themselves; the effect of surprise that Freud could count on when offering an interpretation based in the sexual theory had long since yielded to yawns.

The pass was instituted to mark the termination of a training analysis. Thus it symbolized the passage from the place of analysand to that of analyst. More often than not, someone in training analysis had already begun to receive patients even before termination, so that the pass signified most particularly the renunciation of the position of analysand along with the renunciation of the narcissism inherent in that position. In most cases termination involves an initiative on the part of the analysand; Lacan and the Lacanians looked askance at the practice of the analyst's announcing the end of an analysis. The analysand's initiative to terminate ought eventually to be received and recognized by the analyst.

Once recognized, the analysand could present himself for the pass. The analyst then selected a number of people as potential passers; out of this group the analysand or candidate had to choose two at random. By definition the passers were people in training analysis themselves who were at about the same stage as the candidate. They were the candidate's peers, and there were always two chosen, a pair of peers. Once he had chosen the names, the candidate had to take the initiative of getting in touch with each of these passers in turn. He would talk with the passers for as much time as he felt was necessary to explain to them how he had come to the decision that his analysis was over and how he had decided that he wanted to be a psychoanalyst. So he would tell them his story, the story of his analysis, and, even more important, how he had come to conceptualize his experience.

When the candidate was satisfied that he had explained himself to the passers and that they had understood some-

thing of what he was about, the passers presented themselves on his behalf before a committee, elected from the
membership of the school. The committee decided whether
the candidate should receive a pass or a fail. It had the right
to question the candidate's training analyst and supervisors,
but the point of the pass was that the candidate himself
never went before the committee. He was represented by his
passers. They may have argued either for or against the candidate, and the committee could either accept or reject their
recommendation. Naturally there was always some question
about how the members of the committee could see through
the passers to the candidate.

It is not obvious to me that this procedure should be intrinsically horrifying. Nevertheless it was. First and perhaps
foremost was the idea that the incipient analyst had to talk
about his own analysis, and with total strangers at that.
Since there were many people attempting the pass and since
each of these people had a network of social relations he was
divulging to two people who in turn were divulging it to
eight or so more, the possibilities for the multiplication of
gossip were staggering. To the best of my knowledge, the
tradition of the professional secret was kept rigorously here.
That is not really the question. The problem was that people
felt they were in some sense being compromised by this request to tell about their analysis, and since the Ecole was a
place where conflicting passions often led to wars, who knew
when compromising material might be used in one's disfa-
vor?

The answer to this is quite straightforward. There was
nothing in the procedures of the pass that required the candidate to confess his worst secrets. Ultimately, neither the
passers nor the committee ought to have cared at all about
such gossip. It seemed to me that any candidate who presented himself and his analysis in a confessional mode would
have failed the pass.

The second point of opposition concerned the fact that the

candidate could not speak before the committee in his own name, that he could not argue his case, that he had to rely on two people who could be expected to be in a position of rivalry with him, whose motives may not have been the best, and who were no more qualified than the candidate himself. The committee was charged with the task of sifting through the testimony of the two witnesses to get at the real thing, the speaker behind the representatives. While the candidate as subject was in one place, his destiny was being played out in another. Also, it was not so much a question of briefing the passers, of feeding them the right information, of persuading them of the merits of your application. Rather, all things considered, you found yourself faced with the task not of expressing yourself but of tricking the passers into doing your bidding despite themselves. Obviously, this is not a self-evident proposition: it does not state clearly what is going to take place between candidate and passers, between passers and committee. The procedure did not state clearly the criteria for passing and failing. This being the case, one of the few distinctions of the practice of the pass was the amount of anxiety it generated, for the candidates and for those who considered posing their candidacy.

There are of course rationales for this rite. Your destiny is established before you are born in a place you will always consider to be elsewhere. The people who have an influence on that destiny, parents and grandparents, are perhaps people you will never meet or know. Also the position of the analyst is characterized by silence, by coming, one may say, to identify with the position of the silent dead. This does not mean that the analyst cannot talk to his patient, but everything he says will be taken as coming through a filter, as if coming from the dead. The analyst speaks from the place attributed to him in the transference, whether he knows it or not. Why are there two passers? Precisely because signifiers always come in pairs. The subject represents himself with a signifier, and that signifier has as its structure the fact that it is not meaningful except in relation to another signifier. What I mean to say does not necessarily determine what I do say; by now this is almost a psychoanalytic truism.

There is more to the pass than this. The cutting edge of the procedure can best be grasped if we evaluate it in the light of something that has been posited by religion. I think that the horror of the pass, the investment that people placed in the procedure, is only intelligible if we think of it as a psychoanalytic version of the last judgment, with the slight alteration that the pass implies a renunciation of "eternal life." It does not offer rewards, but responsibilities. This version of the act does not correspond in all forms to what happens in Heaven, but the parallels are close enough to make my point. When the time of the last judgment is at hand, whoever is being judged does not have the opportunity to argue his case, to rationalize his acts and words, the conduct of his life. He is not called upon to shed a different light on the history that has been written in what is now a closed book. Whatever tribunal makes the last judgment, the subject does not appear before that tribunal as a living subject. If you must be dead to be judged finally, your past acts and words speak for you. The last judgment is based on acts and not on intentions. Even within the religious forms it makes no sense to say: I intended to live righteously, to repent, but I did not—so judge me by my intentions.

This much said, the last judgment makes no sense to the analysand. The position of the analysand implies that one is analyzing; in French it is always written in the present participle. In English and in some older French theory, the analysand is identified as the one who is analyzed, and Lacan made an important step forward when he declared that analysands analyze. The kinds of things that analysands analyze are generally of no interest in the situation of the last judgment. There no one cares why you did what you did, what childhood factors influenced your ethical courage or cowardice, what determined or motivated you to be what you were.

The tribunal or committee that passes judgment does not analyze your behavior; nor does it analyze the passers. During the course of an analysis people recognize that they have made mistakes in the conduct of their lives; they want to change things so that the same mistakes are not repeated. In analysis one rewrites one's history and learns to act in consequence. While this rewriting is in progress, the analysand renounces responsibility for what has been done, for what has driven him to make an error; he pins it all on someone or something else.

There are many different schools of analysis, and many of them offer different explanations of why things do not work out very well in some people's lives. What differentiates the pass or the passing of judgment from all of these is that, when this point arrives, it no longer matters what factors determined behavior, whether unconscious, environmental, social, cultural, or nutritional. There is a point at which you have to answer for what you have or have not done, for what you have or have not been. And no amount of astute analysis can obviate that responsibility, which is ethical and thus beyond analysis.

At the least this makes clear why people like to do analysis and why the termination of analysis is never anticipated with any great joy. It is more fun, more secure, to analyze than to be in the position of the dead, to be judged in a situation where a heart of gold and all the analytic acuity in the world mean nothing. It is not surprising that people who have strived to be good patients have the greatest difficulty in giving up what it took them so many years to master. And yet is it any more surprising than the gesture of Prospero—abjuring his art and submitting himself to judgment? And doesn't *The Tempest* alert us to the fact that one has to exercise this art before abjuring it, that one has to learn to analyze first if this abjuring is to make any sense? It makes no sense to give up an art that has never been acquired.

During the course of a psychoanalysis the analyst occupies this place of being judged. The analysand's response to the analyst's interpretation renders a judgment on that interpretation. And if that judgment is negative, if the interpretation does not produce the desired effect, it is not a good idea for the analyst to argue about it, to justify himself. During the course of an analysis, the moment of judgment is enacted when the analyst falls silent, fades out of the picture, leaves the analysand's unconscious to its own devices, permits the transference to borrow from him whatever traits it finds useful. If the analyst is to fall silent, this means that at first he has said things, and then becomes silent. The analyst's silence is not a given, it is not his right and privilege, it is not accorded by the fact that he has graduated from an institute. The analyst's silence is earned. He will become like the dummy in a game of bridge, for having pronounced the last pass of the partnership. The dummy must lay his cards on the table, open his hand. One wonders how many analysts put enough cards on the table for the analysand-declarer to play out the hand.

What, then, is so difficult to accept about the pass? Why did it pose such a problem for French analysts when Lacan introduced it? The ethical proposition that one is judged by one's acts and not by intentions or consciousness is not too difficult; we did not need to discover the unconscious to know this. Perhaps it is a sign of the times that people are so enamoured with self-consciousness that any gesture to repudiate it can only be looked upon with fear. Most people would rather dissect or even dismantle their experiences, thus curing themselves of desire. Why is it so difficult for any human being to be in a place that symbolizes death? Is there a way to make the analyst's silence into something that symbolizes sexuality?

It is more comfortable to think that sex is the problem. The question we ask is whether sex signifies life or death. This is a subject of major concern, and also a political issue of considerable dimensions. Freud identified the sexual drives with the life drives; sex mixed with the death drive produces sadism. Like all other perversions, this one is defined in terms of a failure to accomplish an act of heterosexual intercourse. Freud wanted to give sex credit for the production of new life. Once you agree on this point, you not only become agitated about perversions but you become anxious over what are now called sexual dysfunctions. As long as you can accomplish the act of heterosexual intercourse with a reasonable degree of proficiency, you are immune from judgment about sexual performance and, by extension, from judgment about sanity. That the ability to copulate is not clinically a meaningful indicator of much of anything has not shaken people's belief that if they can fuck they are fine: they are judged healthy, with all that implies about the fulfillment of life.

For people who have a stake in thinking that sex signifies life, any sexual act that even hints at a nonprocreative function for sexuality is anathema. And I am not simply talking about sexual perversions, but about any aspects of sexuality that manifest desire. What signifies desire in the sex act are the aspects beyond its accomplishment. To show what this means, take an example from another realm: eating. Lacan said that, even though eating has a basic biological function of nutrition, what you need to nourish yourself has little to do with the way you actually eat. And this is not because people eat the wrong foods; rather it is because the preparation of foods in elaborate configurations, the seeking after a variety of foods and cuisines, the use of good table manners, the taste for Peking duck, none of this has anything to do with nutritional need. Lemon mousse is nourishing, but if your basic interest were nutrition as a life-signifying function, you would be mad to go to the time and expense it takes to acquire a good lemon mousse. The sexual equivalent of the yen for Peking duck or escargots might be considered to be sexual preliminaries, seduction rites, appearance, sexiness, whatever precedes and prepares the act. But we know well enough by now that "being in the mood," desiring sexual activity, is not a given. To develop a yen for sexuality one requires something more than the promise of creating new life. What is important about desire in either case is how to sustain it, how to protract it in time, how to put off the satisfaction of that desire, in order, strangely enough, to make the experience of satisfaction satisfying. The experience of satisfaction is equivalent, as the metaphysical poets said, to dying. Peking duck does not simply satisfy hunger, it satisfies desire, and this is quite a different experience.

So it is death that is desired in eating as well as in the sexual act, and each experience has its way of providing something like the experience of dying. As I said above, the desire for death means that the desire is cultivated to the extent that death is kept at a distance, ultimately to be experienced not as a real death but as *jouissance*, a term that denotes the intense pleasure of orgasm, and other equivalent experiences. When Socrates says that philosophers should practice dying and when Montaigne repeats the same injunction, perhaps they are talking about something that is best done through the exercise of Eros.

Psychoanalysis has traditionally been on the side of life and love; in most schools of analysis the one aspect of Freud's thought that is considered to be a mistake is the death drive. Not without the complicity of Freud himself. In his analysis of Dora, Freud attempts to argue in the most cogent and intelligent fashion that Dora is in love. And he considers his moment of triumph, his pyrrhic victory, the extortion of the admission that his interpretation is correct, that she will no longer resist, that she will, by implication, learn to love and to live. It is hardly coincidental that this moment marks the end of her analysis.

The case is interesting in another respect. It illustrates the problem analysts have in passing from the place of the analysand to the place of the analyst. Doesn't it strike you that Freud, despite my description of the analyst as dummy, talks a great deal? It seems as if he couldn't keep his mouth shut, to take up an analytic position. Why was this so difficult? My opinion is that Freud's interpretations and analyses were so brilliant, so masterful and dazzling, that he simply could not keep them to himself. His mistake was not that his interpretations were wrong but that they were misplaced; they came at times when a sage silence would have been by far the better tactic. Freud could not fade out of the picture symbolically, so Dora had no choice but to fade out of it in reality.

Psychoanalytic and psychotherapeutic theories have come down hard on those who see things in other terms than those of life and the living. Analysts define themselves as life-merchants, their practice as a therapeutic alliance between two living beings or as an interpersonal relationship between living beings. They want to foster an improvement in the way life is lived; they seek empathy between the living. And this is strategically important. Analysts and therapists do not want to be thought of as merchants of despair and morbidity. They talk of growth and development, of the flowering of these natural tendencies. Look at what Erik Erikson says about the pronoun "I"; it has nothing to do with its linguistic function but is transformed into a quasi-mystical affirmation of the value of life: "But 'I' is nothing less than the verbal assurance according to which I feel that I am the center of awareness in a universe of experience in which I have a coherent identity, and that I am in possession of my wits and able to say what I see and think. No quantifiable aspect of this experience can do justice to its subjective halo, for it means nothing less than that I am alive, that I *am* life" (*Identity, Youth, and Crisis*, p. 220).

How can this be related to psychoanalysis when the crux of the analytic situation is the deathlike silence of the analyst? This silence permits the patient to enter into a dialogue with the dead, with his past, not as it lives in memory but rather as it amounts to so many dead letters.

The Greek gods provided a particularly efficacious way of showing the dead as socially relevant. We should not be thrown by the fact that they were called immortal, for immortal simply means not mortal and "not mortal" doesn't always mean living forever or eternally. Not mortal is also a characteristic of the dead. Only the living are mortal. The search for immortality, which we usually interpret as a seeking after eternal life, a wish to deny death, is but another name for the desire for death.

Unfortunately our passion for science and rationality has prevented us from appreciating the role the dead play for the living. The way we reconcile ourselves with the dead, the way we make peace with them, negotiate with them, determines the quality of our experience insofar as we ex-sist, insofar as we are situated in another realm from theirs. We usually think of the dead as phantoms and ghosts, to which no mature adult would lend credence. They become relegated to the world of children, infidels, and savages, these ghosts. But as the affair of children, they come to inhabit the unconscious, and Freud identified the unconscious with the infantile.

Here we can appreciate the importance of Lacan's remark that the gods are real, not imaginary or symbolic. The dead also are real, and not merely because death creates holes in the real. The gods and the dead are real because the only encounter we have with the real is based on the canceling of our perceptual conscious, of our sense of being alive: the real is real whether we experience it or not and regardless of how we experience it. The real is most real when we are not there; and when we are there, the real does not adapt itself or accommodate itself to our being there. The concept of the real implies the annihilation of the subject. When the Greeks named the wind or the sea after a god, they recognized that it is only through the structure of the symbolic order that things become real, not through perception or consciousness, not through the agency of a subject. A subject can only make the real into objects; consciousness can only make it into phenomena.

Through the interaction of consciousness with objects things take on a semblance of reality, but consciousness goes out to encounter the real only on its own terms, in function of consciousness itself. I need not tell you that consciousness has a long and distinguished philosophical history. In general you know that, if you want to increase your consciousness of a petunia, you will concentrate on the form, the color, the location, how you encountered it, the place from which you see it, and so on. And the more you do so, the less it becomes real, the more it becomes . . . a work of art. The petunia is beautiful, and the expansion of consciousness is an aesthetic exercise. The dialogue of consciousness with objects makes these objects into veils, as some philosophers have asserted.

What on earth did Freud then mean when he said that psychoanalysis makes the unconscious conscious? If we accept the fact that many patients have an experience in analysis which resembles their becoming conscious of things they had not been conscious of before, how does this jibe with what I have said about consciousness? Surely analysis does not propose that analysands gain an aesthetic appreciation of the contents of their unconscious!

Hegelian consciousness becomes consciousness of self only to annihilate the self and consciousness with it. The justification for Freud's emphasis on consciousness is that consciousness contains within itself the principle of its own overcoming, its own destruction and simultaneous surpassing. Again we have a kind of passing. The journey of the phenomenology of mind must yield to the science of logic and, if this does happen, the only reason can be that the logic of language subverts the order of consciousness. So consciousness is an aspect of analytic work, but one to be gotten beyond. The principle that makes becoming conscious so satisfying is the same principle that will ultimately subvert consciousness.

Finally, we should not forget that in *The Ego and the Id* Freud said that nothing in the unconscious ever really becomes conscious except as it is translated into preconscious terms; therefore, consciousness only accepts things on its own terms. And when Freud says in "The Unconscious" that all thought takes place in the unconscious, doesn't this tell us that the unconscious is a logic and that it can be known intimately only through the science of logic?

The analyst's place is the place of the dead, in the singular, unnamed. It is for the analysand to name this place, thereby confirming the role of the signifier in its creation. It is not enough for the analyst not to talk; it is impossible for him to remain entirely silent, but when he does talk the analytic situation causes his words to be taken as coming from the dead. The analyst is in the position of the dead whether he likes it or not, whether he accepts it or not. He can do whatever he likes to seem a living breathing human being, a real person, but still his words will be coming from the dead. The only difference is that, in this case, the analyst will be judged as being dead and not knowing it.

For readers of Freud and Lacan this idea should have a ring of familiarity. It refers to a dream Freud analyzed in *The Interpretation of Dreams* and in "Two Principles of Mental Functioning" which tells of a young man, whose father had died, dreaming that his father is talking to him as if he were still alive. The comment in the dream is: he had really died, only he did not know it. Freud interprets this as Oedipal guilt by filling in the ellipses; the father had died because of the dreamer's wish and did not know that his son had wished him dead. The Lacanian addendum to this analysis concentrates on the verb, the implications of the past tense, which in French is rendered in the imperfect (*il ne savait pas*). Lacan says that if he did not know then, perhaps he knows now, or perhaps he will come to know that he is dead. The father must not find out that he is dead because this will render interpersonal relations impossible. Where Freud says that the discovery by a living father of the wish to murder him would have been horrible for the son, Lacan has shifted the emphasis to the relationship with the dead father.

Now, follow Lacan in looking at the aspect of enunciation. Perhaps the dead do talk, but not in the same way as the living. If the dream had come up during an analysis—Freud does not specify that it did—I would read it as a commentary on the analyst's technique, on his ability to know his place, and also as a sign for him to be more faithful to that place. In this situation there is no need for an interpretation or for any other remark that would show that the analyst does not know he is dead. The dream calls for a change in strategy in the conduct of the treatment.

What would this change entail? First, the analyst would have to learn to remain silent, not to interfere in the flow of the patient's associations. Second, and more important, the analyst ought to stop addressing the patient in a conversational tone, stop addressing him as if he were a friend or a social acquaintance. This is most difficult for analysts to accept or to act on. A change of tone and a change in the construction of the sentences that the analyst pronounces—making them more incisive and decisive, for example—these are the kinds of interventions that will be helpful here. And they will be far more helpful than any interpretation of the dream. Whereas an interpretation tends to offer a meaning or even an explanation, a change in tactics or strategy affords the analysand the opportunity to verbalize the change as he sees fit. More particularly, it will permit him to speak in a situation where the analyst's speech is acting as a resistance. And when we say that the analyst's speech is acting as a resistance, we mean that his personal presence, his need to be there as a personal presence, is a fundamental point of resistance in analysis. It is crucial in the conduct of any analysis for the analyst to know when to fade out of the picture.

And this is precisely what is in question in Lacan's invention of the pass. Because the passers go before the committee in place of the candidate, the personal presence of the candidate ought not to exert undue influence on the committee's deliberations. The candidate for the pass has been called upon to show not that he can speak in his own person, but that he can speak through others, from another place. This is not the same as to say that the candidate will make his passers into his mouthpieces, simply expressing what he would have said were he there in person. The passers are not there to tell the candidate's story. What they will tell is the effect of his story on them. And the committee will judge whether this candidate is an Orlando still pining for the love of his Rosalind, whether he is a Lear railing against the universe and his ungrateful daughters, or whether he has reached the state I have identified with Prospero. This last state means that he has renounced his narcissism, both the pathological and the normal varieties, that he fully accepts the split between his act of speaking and what is heard of what he has said, that he accepts being in the position of the dead only after his discourse has earned him that position. At this point he will have passed the pass.

5

HOW DID THE PASS COME TO PASS?

Lacan must have asked himself the question: Why would anyone ever become a psychoanalyst? And when the question took this form, Lacan probably thought to himself that he did not have the answer. The question is a simple one, perhaps too simple for us to torture our minds over it, but the answer is far from self-evident. Perhaps Lacan one day, sitting in his analyst's chair, waiting for the next patient, found himself faced with the questions: What am I doing here, how did I get here, and why did I want to be here?

Instituting a ritual was Lacan's way of posing this question for others, asking them to respond to it. Lacan never promoted himself as having the answers. At best he was a questioner, at times acting like a Zen master, becoming himself a splendid enigma. Within the confines of his theory this place was that of the Other, the capital Other or the grand Other. Those he called his students felt themselves obliged to respond, to offer answers, most of which this Other found not entirely satisfying. They were encouraged to offer better answers, because after all there is a way of responding to such questions, a way that acknowledges the desire behind the question and does not attempt to obliterate it.

Most people believe that Oedipus solved the riddle of the sphinx. Certainly Oedipus believed he did, and the people of Thebes in Sophocles' play concurred. The riddle was: What walks on four feet in the morning, two feet in the afternoon, and three feet in the evening? The answer Oedipus offered was *Anthropos*, Man. This destroyed the sphinx and the people saw it as a blessing. Ultimately Oedipus was destroyed, and one might argue that his fate was worse than that of those who had failed to solve the riddle of the sphinx.

What is interesting is that so many people think that Oedipus had the right answer. Perhaps because we are so in love with mankind or because we are impressed by philosophy, we tend not to question whether there may have been a better response. The logic of the answer Oedipus offered is certainly unimpeachable. An infant crawls on all fours, an adult walks on his own two feet, and the old man walks with the aid of a cane. But surely we should be alerted to the fact that defining the riddle in terms of feet bears directly on the history of the protagonist, whose name derives from his swollen feet. What if Oedipus had simply responded: Oedipus. If he had, the play might have taken a different course, and psychoanalysis with it.

Does the riddle bear, as Oedipus thought, on the life cycle of human beings? This is a possible interpretation, but it is not the only one and not even the best one. The sphinx questioned the subject's existence. It challenged Oedipus and the others to question where they had come from and what they were doing there. And the response I have offered—Oedipus, the name, instead of Man, the class—requires nothing more or less than an awareness of the formative role of the signifier in the determination of existence. It is the signifier of the swollen feet that would have provided the clue to a better response, and this signifier is a sympton or a stigma. Oedipus does not recognize it as a signifier and that is his tragedy. For when he discovers that it really is the key to his identity, it is too late.

Being a psychoanalyst implies passing beyond the condition of Oedipus. It also implies placing oneself in discontinuity with the stages of normal human development. The termination of a psychoanalysis is a break with the past or, better, a burial of that past. The book of one's life history, opened by psychoanalysis to be read, is now closed. And the fate of finished books is to be buried or drowned, to follow Prospero here.

Presumably, the analytic candidate at the end of his training analysis is able to tell why he had decided to become a psychoanalyst. He can tell which historical and "neurotic" elements had led him to request a training analysis. But if he has analyzed this, why then does he persist in wanting to occupy the analyst's chair? One answer would be that he identifies with his analyst. This is certainly an important motivating factor, but Lacan thought that an analysis had failed if it ended with the analysand identifying with the analyst. As he saw it, an analysis ends properly when the analysand has exhausted whatever purpose the analyst had served. At the end the analyst is discarded, like a worn and tattered garment. And this is not the same as watching the sphinx heave itself off a cliff. The analysand's act of discarding the analyst is a passing by. When Oedipus answered the riddle of the sphinx, he bypassed the question in as much as that question was himself.

At the beginning of an analysis the analyst is an enigma, a being of desire, whose desire in indefinite. The analyst's desire is not for this or for that; there is no object that can satisfy it. We call it pure desire; it wants . . . but not this or that. In the transference the analysand takes this desire for his own, in the two senses of the word "takes." At first, he believes that it is his own; he sees in the analyst's desire the desire that would be his were he not alienated from it. And eventually he will take this desire away from the analyst, reducing the latter to something like an old rag. At the termination of a psychoanalysis there is no identification of analyst and analysand; the analysand discards his analyst and buries his analysis because he has assumed the Other's desire and has learned to negotiate with a desire that is elsewhere. He no longer desires to continue his psychoanalysis; he wants to get on with things, to reenter the course of things, its discourse.

Before he reaches this point he is involved with the enigmatic analyst through the link we call transference. The transference, as Freud said, is a love relationship. Following Lacan, we consider this love to be passionate. What keeps the couple formed by analyst and analysand together is the passion of the transference. And this passion is based on the fact that the analysand sees in his analyst his own desire, which is obviously something to which he has been attached and which he wants to recover or retrieve, often at any price. When I say that the transference is a passion, I mean that this love ought not to be subsumed under the other forms of love, such as sympathy, concern, empathy, care, or friendship. The difference is that passionate love is Eros and for the Greeks Eros was a god, not an emotion or feeling. As I have been suggesting, there is something inhuman in this enterprise.

If Lacan is right about transference love, and if he is right in saying that this is the motor of the treatment, then the analyst has no business trying to liquidate the transference. Nor has he any business in feeding this passion; paradoxically, the analyst, by accepting a patient into treatment, shows himself willing to tolerate a passion he can neither destroy nor cultivate. Transference love always has an element of reciprocity. The difference between analyst and analysand as far as the transference is concerned is that the analyst retains the exercise of his faculty of judgment, his intellectual faculty, and this permits him to see that this love, when it is most clearly addressed to him, has mistaken him for an other. For emphasis, I mention that a mistake in the identification of the object of the love does not mean that transference love is not love; nor does it mean that the love is false or even that it is a simulacrum of love. Love is real in the transference, it is not just a repetition, and this tells us something that most people know from their own experience: at the height of any passion worthy of the name, there is always a mistaking of the lover for an other.

The fate of the passion of the transference is to burn itself out; probably this is the fate of all passion when it is not fed. The analyst has no business feeding the passion, of acting on it, any more than he has denying its reality. The trick is to permit a desire to rise from the ashes of the transference. And this, you might imagine, is no mean feat. My poorly veiled reference to the story of the mythological phoenix is perhaps too trite to carry the sense I want it to bear. Nonetheless, you can see that if the purpose of psychoanalysis has to do with the recovery of desire, and with it a sense of purpose in life, of knowing what you want and of going out and getting it, then there is no way that desire is going to rise out of friendship, care, empathy, or the like. The road to desire does not pass through *agape* or *philia* or *caritas*. Nor do the proponents of any of these forms of love contend that they lead to a well-founded and well-grounded desire; on the contrary, they generally believe that these forms of love can cure you of desire.

I said that at the termination of a psychoanalysis an analysand knows that his desire is elsewhere. For me, taking the closest example, that elsewhere was the United States. This sounds flat and trivial, but the use of Lacan's conceptual apparatus should in no way exclude such an articulation. When an analysand formulates these things he does not do so in the language of high theory.

Now I will repeat the question I began this chapter with: Why would anyone want to be a psychoanalyst? You notice that this is not the first repetition of the question, and also that I have not yet ventured a response. At the risk of disappointing my reader, especially after such a long buildup, I will say that someone chooses to practice psychoanalysis because he cannot see himself doing anything else, because he cannot think of any other way to deploy his desire in terms of work. For those who choose to practice psychoanalysis, the profession is their "way" in the world, the path they must follow, their Tao.

This is perhaps not very satisfying. Would it be any better to say that people become psychoanalysts because they want to help and to cure others who suffer, because they want to make the world a better place to live in, or even because their own neurotic insufficiencies make them crave the kind of love a patient in the throes of the transference offers to them? These kinds of answers are certainly more conventional, fitting better with what people take to be psychological knowledge. And yet ultimately they do not tell us anything, mostly because they attempt to offer an explanation where in fact no explanation is called for or even required. My response, which I hope will at least seem Zenlike, says that when an analytic candidate finishes his training analysis, if he could think of something else to do with his desire, he would.

Still it takes a certain amount of study to become a psychoanalyst. On the one hand, the training program established by the Ecole freudienne intended to provide an organizational structure that was specifically analytic. On the other hand, the circumstances that led to the founding of the Ecole marked it in such a way as to subvert the analytic process. The school was founded after Lacan was excommunicated from the International Psychoanalytic Association. Lacan and his teaching were thus stigmatized, one might even say cursed, by Freud's heirs, and the Ecole freudienne in my judgment never found a way around this curse. The reaction of the analysts who remained loyal to Lacan was simply to renounce everything that smacked of the methods and approach of the IPA. They tended to make American analysts a collective scapegoat, the repository of conflicts that were tearing their own organization apart. Generally speaking it was good politics to blame it all on the Americans, but the price was high. In making the IPA into a monolith directed from New York, the French analysts were obliged to overlook some interesting and useful discoveries made on the other side of the Atlantic. Even more important, the lack of a dialogue with people who were not believers, who did not share the passionate commitment to Lacan, created an intellectual hothouse in Paris in which everything was related to the Master, whose words were quickly elevated into sacred dicta.

Lacan was instrumental in the establishment of this organization. Eventually, however, he must have grown weary of it, even exasperated. Once upon returning from a trip to America he remarked that only the Americans knew how to question him, meaning that only the Americans were not totally in awe of him and thus they alone challenged his authority with intelligence.

The training program at the Ecole freudienne was never specifically organized. There were no requirements and no formal admissions procedures. Course work was more or less voluntary, and there was no faculty designated as such. Anyone who wanted to offer a course could usually do so. Attendance was open to anyone who wanted to attend—except for some seminars—and there were no fees for attendance. The candidate was required to do a training analysis with an analyst of his choice and to have one or two supervisors. It is not even quite accurate to call the trainee a "candidate"; since there was no formal admissions, the status of candidate meant generally that someone had declared to his analyst and to the secretary of the Ecole that he intended to use his analysis for the purpose of becoming an analyst. Since course work required no examinations or papers—except for an occasional seminar report—you could only think that the decision about your admission as a member of the Ecole rested largely in the hands of your analyst and supervisor. There were boards that decided these matters, but certainly the word of these two people must have had the most weight—outside of the pass, that is. As opposed to American analytic institutes, there was no clinic where candidates could receive their first analytic patients. In the United States these patients are generally screened and referred by the senior analysts who run the clinic. The patients are usually unable to afford to the high fees of experienced analysts, and so they are referred to a candidate who will charge them according to need. Most Lacanians felt that this was a degrading procedure, and Lacan himself had fought to abolish the distinctions between supposedly experienced analysts and those less experienced. More important, all analysts in the Ecole freudienne had a sliding scale that usually began at $10 a session, so there was no question of excluding patients who were less solvent. During the years I was there, an abundance of people wanted to do a psychoanalysis, far outstripping the number of qualified practitioners. Young analysts who had managed to make themselves known did not have much of a problem finding patients. This situation was to change by the late seventies, and certainly the shrinking number of demands for analysis had something to do with the conflicts that emerged then.

The reasoning behind the organization of the Ecole freudienne were as follows. Those who wanted to be a psychoanalyst had to show the initiative and drive to find the courses and study groups that would provide them with an analytic education and also had to make themselves recognized by the others within those groups. No one told you what to do or where to go. Steering committees were set up to apprise you of what was available, but there was no organized curriculum and no course requirements that had to be fulfilled. This principle has its sympathetic side: those who declared themselves analytic candidates should be sufficiently adult about it to construct and fulfill their own course of studies, according to what they judged necessary. People were not, in other words treated like children. And rightfully so, since most people who undertake analytic training are in their middle to late twenties. The other side of this situation was that people did not know where they stood. The only real point of certainty was that Lacan and a few other senior analysts had considerable authority and say in the referral of analytic patients and in advancement within the group. This led many people to feel that they had to impress Lacan or to impress someone who was known as a good source for referrals. A well-regarded senior analyst could receive several demands for analysis a week. You might guess that such people were sought out and that many young analysts wanted to work with them, to be their favored students. I am not suggesting that such things do not happen in other analytic institutes; but at the Ecole freudienne things were organized in such a way as to exacerbate ordinary tensions and foster a generalized hysteria that finally led Lacan to dissolve the group.

One aspect of this procedure that American analysts find particularly puzzling is the fact that the wish to become a psychoanalyst was not addressed to a committee of the Ecole but directly to a psychoanalyst and that it had exactly the same status as any other demand for analysis. In this country, if you want to be an analyst you must apply to an institute and go through a screening procedure that assesses your aptness for the profession and your suitability as a future colleague. This filtering process is thought to weed out undesirables, but it is basically a process of exclusion that creates "rejects" who may go to another institute to do their training. Once you are accepted in an American institute, you usually are then recommended to a training analyst. Thus this crucial choice is made for you, and even though you may not want to do an analysis with this person, you can't refuse too many of the committee's selections before you get stigmatized as too resistant. Here one sees the shadow of what used to be called matchmaking: the training analysis in such an institute is an arranged alliance.

Sometimes these alliances work out well for everyone involved. The problem with them is that, if the analysis has as its therapeutic base the establishment of transference love, an arranged alliance is far from the best atmosphere in which to permit such love. There are some who would say that it works in exactly the opposite sense, that it must undermine the transference even before it has begun.

The general feeling in Paris was that love is best when it is unencumbered by bureaucratic rituals, formal requirements, diplomas, graduations, and the other trappings of the university. And if we follow Lacan's relating passionate love to such practices as courtly love, mysticism, or even the passion of Alcibiades for Socrates in the *Symposium*, this is certainly true. The problem was that the Ecole freudienne sustained the passion too well, since its reason for being was the passion people had for Lacan—heretic, pariah,—and it did everything it could to feed that passion. Once the group was dissolved, all one saw in the press and in the salons of Paris was pure passion. Each side tended to blame the dissolution on the other side, defined as those whose passion for Lacan was not true enough. The display, as I have said, did no good at all to the psychoanalytic cause. My personal reaction, reading about the fray through letters, was to stay as far away as possible.

After the dissolution of the Ecole freudienne, one final battle broke out, over the succession. In the midst of it Lacan issued a statement in the form of a letter, and there he said that the question was whether or not his students still loved him. Extraordinary statement, one of the last he made, and its authenticity was immediately disputed by Charles Melman and others who accused Jacques-Alain Miller of having written the letter or of dictating it to Lacan and forcing him to sign it. But the statement, worthy of a King Lear, was not out of character, and it was horrifying to think that this was what the Ecole freudinne had come to or, better, what it had always been.

Miller was also accused of sequestering a sick and frail old man, or refusing to let anyone talk to him, thus of covering up the truth about the authorship of the letter. The tracts stopped just short of accusing Miller of murder, though one I remember vividly attempted through an analysis of Miller's writing to demonstrate that Lacan's son-in-law was comparable to Hitler. The process of scapegoating was repeating itself, only this time it was not against the IPA but against the man Lacan wanted to continue his work. Thus it was directed against Lacan himself in one final paroxysm of Oedipal guilt.

Lacan did attempt to deliver psychoanalysis from its fascination with this paradigm. When he pronounced the dissolution of his school, he echoed the word "dissolution" that appears prominently in Freud in the title of an article, "The Dissolution of the Oedipus Complex." However Lacan, visiting Caracas in July 1980, also declared: "C'est à vous d'être lacanien, si vous voulez. Moi, je suis freudien." Which most took to be a deunuciation of those who called themselves Lacanians. One might say that being a Freudian, insisting on a spiritual and intellectual descendance, had been Lacan's curse and that he did not wish to pass that curse on to his followers.

The Ecole freudienne did not pass the pass, in other words. There were simply too many who believed in Lacan for it to happen. The pass was a ritual, and the introduction of a formal ritual into a group that based its practice on something akin to mysticism, a highly individualized practice that has always defied ritualization and codification, was too much for the group to absorb. Once the question for French psychoanalysis was Lacan the man, once the International Psychoanalytic Association declared that people would have to decide for or against Lacan, the loyal minority, which surely showed the most courage, was struck with a curse—not for having been loyal but for having voted at all, for having even considered the terms of such an outrageous decision. Many felt that they were being forced to believe in Lacan, and this they did. They felt that their powers of judgment had been taken away because any questioning of Lacan was tantamount to betraying him before the IPA. And Lacan accepted what amounted to a sequestering at the hands of those who loved him best; he was, with his full consent, withdrawn from exchange with the worldwide analytic community, with those who refused his teaching and thus became unworthy of any gesture of recognition.

Lacan's complicity was evident in his style, a style that defies translation and is so thoroughly intricated with the peculiarites of the French language that it cannot be rendered in other languages without serious loss. In his later works he uses many Joycean puns, which are totally untranslatable (for example, "hainamoration," "parlêtre"). Also Lacan's construction of a public persona, the importance of his presence, his attitude, his bearing, his dress, even the tone of his voice, as vehicles to understanding his thought made it next to impossible for readers to pick up a text and to evaluate it on its intellectual merits alone, to formulate a judgment outside of an established system of belief. At the same time, Lacan must have known that his reputation and recognition ultimately could only be based on the intellectual content of his work. The problem was that, as a man become almost a work of art, Lacan was the organized center of resistance to his own theories. This provided an impetus for the development of psychoanalysis in France, and it established a base for some exceptionally fine clinical work. There is still a great deal left to be done by Lacanian analysts.

I have offered in this discussion an opposition between judgment and belief, which is not the most usual opposition. Thinkers usually oppose belief with knowledge, thereby opposing religion with science. Roughly, belief and knowledge are both states of mind whereas judgment appears to be strictly an act of the mind. Let me define these terms in relation to psychoanalytic experience.

Belief, in psychoanalysis, relates for the most part to what can be called cures by suggestion. It is well known that some patients will recover remarkably when they believe that their therapist is an accomplished healer. Sometimes a diploma or a title will be enough to establish this authority. In other cases the experience of friends with an analyst will be decisive. In medical practice, belief is the basis for what is called the placebo effect. In some patients psychic economy dictates that it is preferable to give up a symptom rather than to abandon the belief in the ability of the healer. The cure effected by belief is a confirmation of the potency of the healer. Also, it permits the patient to continue to condemn those who did not have the same degree of potency.

Psychoanalysts have always recognized such cures for what they are, imaginary. This does not of course mean that the original complaint was imaginary. The symptom does disappear but analysts have noticed that it is simply displaced, and the patient will return with another malady requiring the ministrations of the healer. The patient who has been cured through belief does not know how he fell ill or why he has been cured. In most cases he does not want to know. And it is probably essential to the structure of a system of beliefs that the believer not want to know what it is that produces these effects. The believer believes that it is the person of the healer that produces the effect, and that is sufficient . . . and satisfying. The justification for the belief is thus not knowledge but rather a state of feeling better. This is taken to be a proof of the power of the healer and of the truth of the healer's beliefs.

Eventually belief becomes firmly grounded or rooted, and it passes beyond doubt. At this point the believer becomes convinced, gains conviction. This does not take place entirely through an act of faith, but is often the result of an experience of cure or of several such experiences. Lacan, for one, stated clearly that psychoanalysis should have nothing to do with states of conviction. In his experience conviction was always associated with the unshakable attitude of psychotics when confronted with any doubt about their beliefs. Paranoics are convinced, and they became for Lacan the very model of conviction.

Thus it is false to say that psychoanalysts are engaged in an activity that will lead their patients to the conviction of the truth of their interpretations. Lacan rejected the idea that, when patients refuse or disagree with an analyst's interpretation, they are resisting and that the resistance should be analyzed. He also never tried to convince anyone to undertake psychoanalysis. That desire must come from the prospective analysand; the most the analyst can do is to offer a treatment.

How then did Lacan see the functioning of interpretation? Imagine an analytic patient who comes to a session and brings material that pertains essentially to his relationship with his mother. Based on what he hears and on his knowledge of psychoanalysis, the analyst may offer a reasonable interpretation. This might be formulated as: the only thing that matters to you is whether or not you are pleasing your mother. Let us imagine that the analysand listens to this and responds that it doesn't seem quite right, that as a matter of fact there was another aspect of the situation, one he thought too trivial to mention, which concerns his father's role in all of this. Taking this new element into account changes the entire picture and makes the interpretation patently inexact.

This process is clearly dialectical, and it works because there is an opposition established, a conflict between patient and analyst. The analyst has simply been had; he's been duped. Some will say that this means that he should not have interpreted at all, but it is clear that his inexact interpretation, firmly grounded in the material he heard, was precisely what permitted the patient to bring forth the new material that gave them both a clearer picture of the structure in question. As Lacan put it, it is essential for the analyst to permit himself to be duped by the unconscious.

The analysand may then formulate a new interpretation in which it is not he who was concerned with pleasing his mother but his father who wanted to please his wife and who never seemed to be adequate to the task. Now the analysand sees that the path to his own identification with his father has been blocked and, with it, his gaining a sense of his own masculinity. The question of his existence is posed from the place he is obliged to occupy in his family, given the problems that define his parents' marriage.

This is a well-enough known paradigm for an obsessional neurosis. When the subject has understood this and articulates it—preferably in opposition to his analyst—then we say that he has gained insight or awareness. Now Lacan was not totally satisfied with these terms and used the broader term of "knowledge" to describe what the subject has acquired—or even has stolen.

What takes place here is of the order of theft. Often enough analysands say that they are being ripped off by their analysts, that the fee is too high and they are not getting enough for their money. This is a response to the idea that knowledge is bought by the analysand, that there is some kind of equitable exchange taking place. Here I would refer you to Norman O. Brown's *Hermes the Thief* where the transactions presided over by Hermes are described as mutual thievery. The reason is that the person with whom exchange is entered into is defined as a stranger, an Other, and there is no possibility of mutually satisfying exchange with such a person. One can never be sure of what the Other wants or whether the Other is satisfied. Thus the statement made by analysands labeling their analysts as thiefs is true; even Lacan said that psychoanalysis was an *escroquerie* (swindle). But that is only half a truth; the other half is that the analysand himself is also a thief—he can never know the true price of the knowledge he gains. Or, better, that price never corresponds to the value.

What is this knowledge? Earlier we saw that the analyst's interpretation disengaged a structure that could be stated as a proposition. For Lacan, knowledge is something that is written as a logic. The key to understanding the unconscious is to see that it is structured logically. One of the great discoveries of psychoanalysis was that this logic defines the strange behaviors of the neurotic. When a patient says that his actions are irrational, that there is no rhyme or reason to what he has become, then we say that he does not want to know.

A neurosis can be written down as a series of formulas like the one I gave for obsessional neurosis. And the process through which these formulas emerge with clarity into the mind can also be written down as a series of logical transformations. This is not at all the same thing as finding the meaning of the symptoms or the meaning of life. The knowledge articulated by psychoanalysis does not make life more meaningful. The neurotic, we can say, is inhabited by meanings he ignores. Bringing these meanings into consciousness does not provide relief from the symptoms unless they lead to the acquisition of knowledge.

Lacan wanted to formalize the structures of psychoanalysis. By this he meant writing them in the kind of letters that have been the hallmark of formal logic since the time of Aristotle's *Organon*. Certainly such a project could not cover the entirety of the field, nor was it intended to. But if such a logic can be developed, following the example Freud established in "A Child Is Being Beaten," then this knowledge cannot as such become a true object of consciousness. It is only grasped fully when it is written.

Here I am saying nothing more than what Freud said in "The Unconscious" and in *The Ego and the Id* when he declared that the materials of the unconscious could not be present to consciousness without passing through preconscious word-representations. If the thing-representations in the unconscious are ultimately readable as letters, as forming letters, these letters can only become clear to consciousness when they are part of words. As such they gain a meaning that is the meaning of the words, and consciousness will latch onto those words as the content of the unconscious. A child sees a woman's legs spread in the form of an M or a V, and if the experience makes a sufficient impression, this letter will run through his history as a thread linking the names of people and places, each of which will take on a certain meaning for consciousness. And as far as consciousness is concerned, this meaning will be sexual. That the inscription of a letter in the unconscious happens in a traumatic experience means nothing more or less than that the body seen as a letter is fixed, immobile, and thus dead.

Let us say, then, that through the course of a psychoanalysis the analysand acquires knowledge about the structure of his symptoms. Is this in itself enough to make him let go of his symptoms, to change the way he relates to whatever he has to relate to? Here the answer is no. Our discussion of interpretation and the theft of knowledge tells us that it is of capital importance that the subject have this knowledge as something that is his. This requirement is also covered by the idea that the knowledge should be writeable. And yet how often we have heard people say that they know exactly what is wrong with them, they have learned all the causes, and still it hasn't changed things in any appreciable way.

Having knowledge is not inconsequential, as we know through Faust. But there has to be an active function, which I will call the function of judgment, that will permit the subject to make his way—assuming that it is *his* way—not according to what he knows, but rather according to what he wants. Lacan was categorical on this point, which is the topic of the better part of his unpublished seminar "The Ethics of Psychoanalysis." The fate of the knowledge acquired through psychoanalysis is to be surpassed. This is what is in question in the pass. The analysand when he finishes his analysis ought to put it behind him; most analysts know this well. If someone has finished a psychoanalysis and still spends much of his time thinking over the experience of the analysis, mulling it over, the analysis has not been very successful.

Thus the termination of a psychoanalysis involves a judgment on the part of the analysand that it is over and that he must act to leave. Certainly the analyst has a role to play here, in acknowledging the correctness of the judgment, in not refusing the analysand's desire to take his leave. This is a recognition by the analyst that the analysand's desire is elsewhere. Through judgment the mind or intellect is engaged in deciding one way or the other. A judgment has to go one way or the other; exercising it a subject declares which one is his way.

References to judgment are rife in psychoanalytic writings. Did Freud, as some have suggested, destroy the innocence of childhood, or was he trying to relieve people of their guilt about sexuality? Is the label of neurosis or psychosis a judgment on the part of the analyst or psychiatrist? When an analyst accepts someone for a psychoanalysis, is he therefore judging that person as sick? Lacan was judged by the International Psychoanalytic Association as unfit to teach and train analytic candidates. What was the effect of this judgment on those who were in training analysis with him? How many people began their careers under the shadow of this condemnation? And when the IPA said that those who had trained with Lacan and who then agreed that he was incompetent could be instated as full members, was it not offering redemption for those who showed themselves to be sufficiently repentant? The authority that judged guilt could also be sufficiently generous to exculpate and exonerate. At a price, of course.

I would be remiss not to mention here the moral strictures

of the superego whose harsh judgments create guilt and remorse. Nor should we forget the theory of object relations
with its division of the world into good and bad objects,
good and bad parenting. Assigning fault for neurosis and
trauma has been almost endemic to psychoanalytic thinking,
though the best analysts have always been uneasy about the
moralizing tone that pervades the literature. The concept of
judgment concerns making distinctions, in the sense of assigning values. Perhaps more important, the act of judgment
engages a dialectic between the one who judges and the
other who is judged.

Hegel wrote of the "beautiful soul" who denounces the
world in order to maintain a personal sense of moral purity
and innocence. Others refuse to pass judgment because they
are most comfortable when they are submitted to judgments, especially when that judgment condemns them as
guilty. These extreme cases represent a polarization intended to cancel the dialectic of judgment. This dialectic is
structural. The phrase "to pass judgment" as used in everyday language implies that I pass judgment on an Other. If I
want to make a judgment concerning myself, I must first
take that self as an Other. This is perfectly consistent with
what Lacan said about desire. His point was that I always
find my desire outside of me because what I desire is always
something that I lack, that is other to me. However, judgment should lead to action, and I should act according to my
desire. For me to act according to a desire that I have found
in an Other I must first have judged that that Other's desire
is mine. The idea that the Other's desire is good or bad does
not enter Lacan's thinking. The dialectic then determines
the identification of a desire as mine where the subject who
judges is not the Other who desires. The subject who desires
is always an other subject. Once the judgment is made, I act
and that act, determined by the judgment of desire, is not
superseded by the act. The desire I judge to be mine is not
discovered by feeling or intuition; it never becomes a func-

tion of Self, and there is never an absolute certainty that it is mine. The action taken does not resolve the splitting of the subject; it enacts it.

To elaborate this concept of judgment as it is applied within psychoanalysis, I will refer to a short paper by Freud entitled "Die Verneinung" or "Negation" (found in the Standard Edition, XIX, 235-239). Lacan's discussion of it is contained in two articles published in his *Ecrits*.

Here is one of Freud's definitions of judgment from the paper: "Judging is the intellectual action which decides the choice of motor action, which puts an end to the postponement due to thought and which leads from thinking to acting." The judging subject is one who acts in the world according to a decision he had taken. When a subject is burdened with an overbearing sense of guilt, when he broods obsessively about crimes real and imaginary, his mental activity is a function of thought and not of judgment. The subject feels himself judged, not judging; the reason for wanting to be judged is to idealize a judge who could not have made a mistake.

Perhaps it is somewhat surprising to find Freud talking of judgment in a paper that concerns the logical function of negation. (We will do better to follow the French authors here and call it denegation, thereby distinguishing it from other forms of negation and bringing it closer to the idea of denial.) The *Verneinung* is a negation that denies something. What it denies is precisely an element from the unconscious that has found its way into an articulated sentence. Freud's examples show this clearly. A patient declares: "Now you'll think I mean to say something insulting, but really I've no such intention." Or, "You ask who this person in the dream can be. It's *not* my mother." Denegation permits the speaking of unconscious material that would otherwise be censored by the ego. The subject says, "This is not me or this is not mine," but he also says, "This is yours." Thus denegation, from a Lacanian perspective, affirms the existence of an

Other with whom the subject wishes to maintain his difference. And the Other is not defined as possessing wisdom; on the contrary, the subject who uses a denegation says that what the Other is supposed to be thinking is precisely wrong. Not only is the Other out there, different from the subject, but he is mistaken.

Freud goes on to say that there are two sorts of decisions for judgment to make. The first is the *Bejahung*: "It affirms or disaffirms the possession by a thing of a particular attribute." The second is the *Verneinung*: "it asserts or disputes that a presentation has an existence in reality." The *Bejahung* is then expressed by Freud in the language of the oral phase, where it refers to what the child wants or does not want to eat, what he wants or does not want to become part of himself. The attribute is "good to eat."

Knowing that something is good to eat is obviously not enough. The subject must also judge whether the thing possessing this attribute is out there in the real world. This has been called reality testing, but it is clearly not at all like the idea that when I walk down the street I can tell whether the fire hydrant I see is real or not. An object that may or may not be found in reality is, as Freud says, one that provided a "real satisfaction" but has been lost. Thus he declares that it is not so much a question of finding an object as of "refinding" it, "to convince oneself that it is still there."

The function of denegation tells us that objects in the world are real, not as a function of the ego's perceptions but as a function of a judgment that defines them in terms of otherness. And this is neither good nor bad, since the categories of good and bad are part of the function of *Bejahung*: good-to-eat or bad-to-eat. When the subject declares that the analyst must be thinking something but that it is certainly not true, and when we say with Freud that whatever has been negated in the sentence is the unconscious material, are we not saying that the subject experiences the unconscious as what Lacan called "the discourse of the Other"?

At times Lacan identified the Other with the death drive. And Freud at the end of his paper says that denegation belongs to this same drive. The judgment of affirmation or belonging, the *Bejahung*, he declares to be a function of Eros. Denegation, he continues, belongs to the destructive drive. This is simply another way of saying that the material of the unconscious is stolen from the dead. And when an analysand says that the analyst must be thinking something or other but that he is wrong, the articulation of unconscious material is shown to be stolen from the analyst, who is in the place of the dead because he is silent. When the anaysand says that it is not what the analyst thinks it is, has he not been caught red-handed with the product of his theft in his hands? Through denegation he says that what he is saying is not his; nor does he want it to be his. The analysand would like to send the unconscious material back whence it came. He uses denegation to protest his innocence, usually in vain. He wants nothing to do with this Other who puts words in his mouth, words that are not his.

So much does he want nothing to do with the Other that the analysand falls in love with it. Through the passion of the transference the analysand will identify with the good traits of the analyst, will borrow them to become like the analyst. Imitation is said to be the most sincere form of flattery, but Freud is telling us that access to the unconscious is blocked by this effort to make the Other into one of us. And this is why Lacan finally rejected identification of the analysand with the analyst as a satisfactory conclusion to an analysis.

The fate of the material that fell under the symbol of negation is not to be assimilated. It will always retain a quality of otherness, and analysts should not try to have their patients integrate it. To use other terms, the fire stolen from the gods ought not to be assimilated as passion or fever; it ought ultimately to be deployed or used—and why not for cooking? The initial product of the act of theft is knowledge, as the myth of Adam and Eve states unambiguously. And it is only through judgment that action will come to pass in which this fire is instrumental. This is the way of existence.

The function of denegation determines the existence of things in the world, "whether it is there in the world, so that he can get hold of it whenever he needs it," as Freud says. The existence of things is one thing, but the subject's ex-sistence is quite another. What interested Lacan ultimately was not the subject's assimilation of love objects, but rather the subject's gaining of ex-sistence. And this must imply an ability to occupy the place of the Other, not in the sense of identifying with someone who is taken to be one's counterpart or little other, but rather in this sense: having appropriated something that does not properly belong to the living, the analysand finds himself detached from humanity and the life cycle. But he is also away from the place of the dead from which he has stolen speech. Now he emerges from the protracted sleep of analysis, not to luxuriate in being but to face the real and perhaps to act according to his desire.

If this is where a psychoanalysis ends, why would anyone want to do it?

6

WHY IN THIS DAY AND AGE DOES ANYONE WANT TO GO through psychoanalysis?

In New York the heyday of Freudian psychoanalysis was the 1950s. Since then more and more people have been choosing therapy over analysis. Everyone seems to be "in therapy." Add to that the growing recourse to medication—both licit and illicit—and psychoanalysis in New York has been confronted by a larger number of mental health "consumers" of which the great majority does not want to do a psychoanalysis.

When I was in Paris, psychoanalysis was growing by leaps and bounds. Alternate therapies were unheard of and medication, while in use, had not cut into the market for analysis. Being in analysis was a badge of honor, and people within the community had full confidence that, no matter how badly the analysis seemed to be going, the skilled analyst would manage to set things right. The absorption of psychoanalytic knowledge, mainly through the influence of Lacan, had produced a state of inebriation in educated Parisians; an intellectual and social ferment swept through the city.

After the dissolution of the Ecole freudienne and the attendant wretching, the psychoanalytic community found itself with a bad hangover. All of a sudden there were far fewer demands for analysis, except for those whose practices were well established. And people began considering alternate therapies for the first time. Was this simply a repetition of the situation Americans had already lived through?

One of the reasons for the growth of psychoanalysis in Paris was that it was affordable to a significant segment of the population. During the 1970s the average fee for a psychoanalytic session in Paris was between $10 and $20. By the end of the decade it had moved up a notch, but it was still far less expensive than a session in New York, which was running at the time between $60 and $100. One of the reasons analysis fell out of favor in the United States is that the analysts priced themselves out of the market. They felt themselves obliged to do so because, according to the senior New York analyst, Jacob Arlow, they wanted to maintain a standard of living roughly equivalent to that of their medical school classmates. The other reason was that the fifty-minute hour limited them to around eight patients a day. In Paris the Lacanians could see two or three patients an hour and thus were not obliged to charge fees that restricted analysis to those who were either rich or had very good insurance. (This was the economic consequence of Lacan's introduction of short sessions, which I will discuss in the next chapter.)

Psychotherapy defies generalization. The term is an umbrella that covers such diverse practices as art therapy, primal-scream therapy, behavioral modification, sex therapy, psychoanalytically oriented therapy, institutional psychotherapy, phobia clinics, EST, transcendental meditation, family therapy, peer-group counseling, ergotherapy, jogging, hot tubs, and dope. For those seeking help there is a veritable embarrassment of riches. The choice of a therapist is not merely the consequence of which mode appeals to the prospective patient. Some of these therapies specialize in particular problems, and within some of the others there are therapists who themselves specialize. The move toward specialization is justified by the idea that there is a treatment of choice, as defined by the relevant manual.

Psychotherapy concerns the problems of living. The therapist directs his gaze at a specific problem and considers his therapy successful if that problem is eliminated. Often the therapist expects that his patients will finish therapy being happy or successful or fulfilled in whatever sense these terms are meaningful to him. Sometimes the patient will need to learn how to be happy, but otherwise it is assumed that, if his symptoms and problems are dealt with effectively, then he will naturally be happy and more productive.

The subspecialty called individual psychotherapy owes the most to psychoanalysis. The difference would appear to be that therapy focuses on specific problems and that the therapist is not a silent enigmatic figure, but a living human being, at times almost a friend who will help patients through the difficult moments of their lives, arranging with them their social and work relations. The therapist accentuates what is positive in the patient's life and tries to separate out what is negative, anxiety-provoking, depressing, or what have you.

Presented in this way, therapy is enormously appealing. Existing within a specific social context and responding to the conscious needs of the members of the group, psychotherapy is a practice that is oriented toward the consumer. It is made to sound like a service whose consumers are as normal as anyone else. Psychotherapy has become a part of everyday life, and in all likelihood it produces some positive results. It rarely engages in high theory because results are its justification for being. In this sense it does not differ very much from other systems of belief that offer positive gains as far as living one's life is concerned.

Usually, the base of psychotherapy is psychology as a science. A lot of therapy may not sound very scientific, but since most of it is practiced by psychologists and psychiatrists, there is a clear presumption that the practitioners *know* something and that what they know can be demonstrated scientifically, according to accepted procedures of evidence and proof. One of the reasons that therapy chooses to treat specific problems is that thereby the results can be measured and the effectiveness of the treatment proven.

It is essential here to note a point Bruno Bettelheim recently made (*The New Yorker*, March 1, 1982). He said that when Freud related psychoanalysis to psychology, it could not have crossed his mind that psychology was a behavioral science. For Freud psychology was a branch of philosophy. Modern psychotherapy has something of a split personality. On the one hand it professes to offer care, concern, help, success, and happiness, as if it were a secular religion. On the other, its practitioners are men and women of science, people who know and who will impart their knowledge to those in need. Behind the enterprise is the belief that the more you know the happier and more successful you will be, that knowledge is a good, perhaps even the supreme good, and that it is capable of solving human problems.

The price is the compartmentalization of the human psyche, its division into discrete and treatable parts. If this were the only payment required, there would probably be no objections raised to these procedures. Yet we know that there have been objections, even some serious ones, about the fact that the treatment and cure of an isolated symptom may generate other symptoms that are disregarded because they are outside the ken of the therapist. And there are studies that have suggested that spending six months on a waiting list is more therapeutic than six months with a competent therapist. I might even add that the idea that scientific knowledge is intrinsically good has been vigorously debated within the community of scientists. The values of happiness and success as proofs of the effectiveness of a therapeutic process have been questioned and perhaps even refuted by the legend of Faust. What this legend shows, among other things, is that finite results, curative as they may be, are nothing compared with the transfinite price that has to be paid somewhere down the road.

In any case I do not mean to engage in the debate over whether psychotherapy is good. Since it seems more correct to talk about therapies, in the plural, I would simply note that psychotherapies are promoted and presented by their practitioners as goods. The reason for this discussion is to sustain the question I began this chapter with: Why in this day and age does anyone want to go through psychoanalysis?

Lacan had very little to say about psychotherapy and psychology. The path they followed was not his. His favorite interlocutors were not academic psychologists, but the luminaries, as he called them, of the past: Aristotle, Hegel, Kant, Socrates, Shakespeare, Sophocles. This strategy intended to place psychoanalysis in the line developed by these luminaries, to make it into a discipline that commanded respect not only for what it was and what it could do but also for the intellectual heritage that gave it sustenance.

Lacan tended to dismiss scientific psychology as alien to his enterprise, as a product of what he saw as the worst tendencies of American life. He thought that the basic inspiration of American psychology was behavioristic, and he joined most analysts in finding this appalling. The question he asked from time to time about behavioristic experimentation was why anyone would want to run these experiments—a question of the desire of the experimenter.

This kind of categorical dismissal was characteristic of Lacan, except when it came to those he considered luminaries. He would probably have agreed with Nietzsche's dictum that we have more to learn from the errors of great minds than we do from the truths of small minds. This kind of haughtiness runs against our grain, and lumping psychology entirely under the category of behaviorism is facile and untrue. There is and there will continue to be much in psychology that can instruct psychoanalysis. Doubtless Lacan knew this; if his work did not permit him to enter into any sort of fruitful dialogue with psychology, surely he had other reasons.

These reasons are not difficult to find, nor are they mysterious. Lacan believed in the classics; he was outraged to see that the passion for science and for scientific knowledge was in the process of producing generations of psychologists and psychoanalysts who had no idea whatsoever of intellectual history, who had never studied Descartes or Spinoza because they were spending their time setting up experiments to prove or disprove some point whose validity was relevant only within the terms of the experiment. Perhaps there is nothing intrinsically evil about data, but the point Lacan wanted to make was that the conclusions drawn from experiments, to say nothing of the hypotheses that animate them, are only as good as the concepts the experimenter has at his disposal. There is no doubt about Lacan's success in this area. Thanks to him, several generations of French psychiatrists, psychologists, and psychoanalysts were well read in the classics—not simply because they had taken a course or two in philosophy, but because the study of philosophy and literature became an ongoing enterprise for the considerable number of people who followed Lacan's teaching, regardless of whether or not they were Lacanians.

When it came to saying something about the reasons that lead a person to do a psychoanalysis, Lacan knew that it was not the wish to be normal, not the wish to be informed of the latest experimental results or the wish to adapt to the environment or the wish to have another caring and concerned friend, that led people to his door. The image of the psychoanalyst as Lacan embodied and cultivated it was that of a disciplined madness, a divine but controlled lunacy. Lacan's analysands were in no way expected to identify with that position, but it is certain that people in Paris were fascinated, enthralled, and scandalized by the grandeur of this Other. Lacan's desire was so intrinsically perplexing that one could not help being perplexed by one's own desire. He was so far from any ideal of a responsible, respectable pillar of the community that people could see that he desired and that he acted according to his desire.

Even in the beginning, when Freud was discovering psychoanalysis, there were many cases of people who presented themselves at the analyst's doorstep as a last resort. Today when all else has failed, when the promises of therapy have faded, when hope has been abandoned, when people have nowhere else to turn, often enough they will call a psychoanalyst. This is a dramatization that may not be precisely true, but it does show us that psychoanalysis has always been considered different from all other forms of therapy. As long as Lacan had anything to say about it, analysis in France jealously guarded this status.

Undertaking a psychoanalysis is not simply a normal part of a normal life. It should not be done for the fun of it, out of curiosity, or to pass the time of day. Not only should it not become part of a daily routine, but it should not in itself be conducted in a routine fashion, as if the analyst were simply repeating a tried and true laboratory experiment. People do not come to psychoanalysis to learn the theory of the unconscious; they seek some knowledge of their own unconscious insofar as that unconscious is particular to them, is singular. And this is where scientific procedures seem to fall short. The scientific truths of psychology concern classes and categories of people within specific situations that are measurable. If human experience is not measurable, if a part of it does not show up in the data, the psychologist may arrogantly assume that it does not exist. Analysts know well that the best interpretations are not those that echo some bit of knowledge gleaned from a textbook. Instead they speak to the analysand as a singular subject. When psychology defines normal stages of human development and when therapists attempt to make sense of their patients' experience by referring them to some putative normality, what they are doing is finding a convenient place for their patients within the concept they have of humanity. They teach their patients to identify with mankind. This is another identification that patients in analysis do not seek and should not be encouraged to develop. Such an identification is nothing more or less than the repression of subjectivity, of personal style, of quirks and idiosyncrasies.

People who present themselves for psychoanalysis are said to be alienated from the norm. Perhaps this is true, but that does not justify attempting to reinsert them in that norm. They are alienated because they have had a taste of something else, and once they have had that experience the norm does not seem to be worth the bother. Analysands, and not only Lacanians, often say that they do not want to become part of normal life because it strikes them as insufferably boring. Their problem is not that they are alienated from the norm, but that they have considerable difficulty in dealing with normal people. The fact that one chooses not to follow the same rules as everyone else is one thing; being unable to deal with the reality of normal people is quite another.

The neurotic's human relations are determined by his dealings with his ghosts. This is not resolved by attempts to exorcise or vaporize these ghosts in bringing the neurotic into intimate contact with some kind of life force or developmental cycle. The neurotic does not get along with his ghosts, does not know how to deal with them, tries to forget them. The value of his experience is precisely that he retains a sense of the existence of the ghosts, the dead, while others succeed admirably in forgetting them.

Ordinarily the social order has myths and rituals that permit its members to make peace with the dead, with ancestors. If the neurotic tries to accomplish the same thing as an individual, showing himself and all individuals taken as individuals to be unequal to the task, this certainly suggests that society has failed in its task of symbolizing death for its members. We might say that the relationship between any subject and the symbolic order always contains the possibility for failure; the human subject as singular being is not after all a symbol. Or else, we could say, changing the mode, that total success here is impossible. So if the members of a social group begin to show signs of neurosis with frequency, this suggests that society has given up on the project of finding a symbolization for death and the dead. Call this a cult of the individual or a worship of the life force, of health, of youth; it is basically a belief in the power of the imaginary to release us from the symbolic.

A person who sees an analyst is seeking a therapist who will not meddle in his life. Paradoxical as it may seem, the analysand is not looking for advice about how to live his life; he does not want to know what the analyst would do in the same situation, and he does not expect the analyst to be his friend or confidant. Basically the analysand wants his analyst to mind his own business, to be interested in the things that concern him, directly or indirectly. And the analyst's business is the transference.

The reason that anyone consults a mental health professional is suffering. What he asks for is relief from this suffering; his demand is for a cure. Lacan, who was so meticulous in distinguishing demand from desire, said that what he demands is surely not what he wants. An analysis does not begin with the analyst promising a cure or even suggesting that in most cases of the same sort a cure is something that can be expected. The question of the beginning of a psychoanalysis is whether the analyst accepts or refuses the patient's suffering. A therapist who applies himself singlemindedly to the immediate task of relieving suffering is refusing that suffering and his patient with it. When I talk of accepting suffering, I mean quite simply that the analyst ought to recognize the validity of the experience of suffering. It is not a foreign element in the patient's life, but essential to the patient's existence. Suffering is the existence the neurotic knows and is not something to be rejected as sick, therefore only valid as it gives the therapist an occasion to practice his trade.

This is not to say that the analyst derives any particular pleasure from the suffering of his patients or that he does not care whether they suffer or not. Nor does it mean that there are no limits to how much suffering is tolerable by an analysand. No analyst is entirely oblivious to these facts, and none considers suffering to be intrinsically good. So when the analyst accepts his patient's suffering, this also means that he permits himself to be implicated in whatever it is that has produced that suffering—this through the transference, which Lacan said was something that analysts have to suffer, as a passion.

An analysis begins with an act, the act by which the analyst accepts someone as an analysand. This is an act of recognition, of the recognition of desire, because the desire of the neurotic is implicated in his suffering. Press forward too quickly to eliminate the suffering and the desire will be eliminated with it. Certainly the fact that the analyst recognizes the validity of the experience of suffering, and thereby recognizes the analysand as desiring, makes the suffering more bearable. Otherwise no one would continue an analysis when it is clear that psychoanalysis cannot in most cases provide relief from symptoms with anything like the rapidity of an injection of Valium.

I am of course speaking of suffering as an existential state, not as the consequence of a physical ailment. There was an interesting case written up in Paris at the time I was there which seems to run counter to what I have just said. The author of a book entitled *Les Mots pour le dire* (The Words To Say It), Marie Cardinal wrote of the beginning of her analysis in the following terms. She had for some time been afflicted by uterine hemorrhaging. Her physicians had tried many different remedies in vain. Finally they decided to operate. Cardinal agreed and checked into a hospital. But as the time of the operation approached she had second thoughts and wanted as a last resort to try psychoanalysis. So she got out of her bed, dressed, and went to see a psychoanalyst. She told him the story of her symptom, and he said nothing except that he wanted to see her the next day. The next day she returned ready to continue talking about her bleeding. As soon as she broached the topic, the analyst stopped her and requested that she talk about something else. She complied with his request, changed the subject, and completed her session. The next morning when she awoke she noticed that the bleeding had stopped. At the time of her writing the book approximately eight years later, she could say that this abnormal hemorrhaging had not returned. What did continue for several more years was her analysis. Thus what we see is a special case of the beginning of a psychoanalysis.

The symptom, however, was not neurotic, but psychosomatic. And as much as this might resemble faith healing, there is in this incident something that is properly psychoanalytic. Through the gesture of prohibiting discourse on the bleeding, the analyst was saying something and what he was saying obviously made sense to the patient. All of this took place and produced an effect without the patient's being able to verbalize what happened. We can even ask whether the analyst at the moment of his intervention could have said what he had to say otherwise, or whether he found the simple gesture of introducing a break or a cut to be the most effective.

What did the analyst say? Simply: You do not need to have a physical symptom to talk to me. Moreover, since I am a psychoanalyst and not a physician, the subject of your speech is you and not your symptom. The suffering that brings you to my door is not the pain of the psychosomatic symptom, but that of being deprived of all forms of speech that do not take this symptom as their subject. Thereby the analyst accepts the patient's suffering and does not state that his intention is the immediate elimination of the illness. Quite the contrary, he is telling her that psychoanalysis is not directed toward the suffering of illness but rather toward something that is called psychic or even existential suffering.

Perhaps this gives more substance to one of Freud's great gestures in founding psychoanalysis: his idea that there ought to be no prearranged topic for sessions, that the patient should simply talk about whatever came to mind. All analysts follow this rule assiduously, but note that in the case of the psychosomatic symptom it is more the principle than the rule itself that is applied.

It is too strong to say that the analyst restores the patient's speech. All the analyst can do is offer to the patient access to speech. This speech, being described as free association, is not centered on a particular subject; the only subject the analyst recognizes is the subject of the unconscious. There may be some confusion over the differing uses of the word subject here. On the one hand I use it to refer to the topic of conversation, but on the other I talk of the subject as the one who is speaking. This kind of equivocation was very dear to Lacan, and he always tried to accentuate it. To eliminate it would be to label the speaking subject the Self, which should be avoided. What we want to do is to grasp the fact that the equivocation is not gratuitous or fatuous. If we are willing to question it, it will tell us something that perhaps we did not know before: when the symptom is the subject of the discourse, then the symptom is speaking. To put it another way, the patient in that case is spoken by the symptom, and when this happens the patient is effectively deprived of her speech insofar as that speech can function to give her access to a desire that would be hers. As the bearer of a symptom, the subject is prey to someone else's desire.

She ignores this desire as well as the identity of the someone else.

So that there should be no confusion, I do not mean to offer the example of Marie Cardinal as a criticism of medical practice. Her physicians were acting according to the most responsible medical ethics, which dictates that they stop the bleeding. The bleeding may have a significance or a meaning for the patient, it may be invested in some particular way historically, but this the physician ignores, by definition. He also ignores the significance that bleeding has within social rituals, not the least of which is the ancient medical practice that prescribed bleeding for all manner of ailments. Physicians can act in a thoroughly professional way ignoring all of this, and generally they do. One does wish, however, that they would be more modest in their claims for their practice. Surely Marie Cardinal could have been cured of her uterine hemorrhaging by a hysterectomy, which would have put a stop to the bleeding. Similarly, there is no doubt that techniques like behavioral modification cause symptoms to disappear. I do not think it is too much to expect from those who practice such arts that they open their ears to other things that are being said to them.

Psychoanalysis bars all but the speaking subject, according to the rule of free association. This encourages the analysand to engage in a kind of verbal incontinence that in itself is an extremely pleasurable activity. Free association is precisely what you do not do in normal conversation—at least not if you wish to continue having normal conversations. It is certainly a discipline, since it requires that the analysand say anything that comes to mind without regard for the relevance of the remark or for whatever pain its articulation may produce. This discipline is acquired slowly and with difficulty; it is extremely rare that an analysand knows how to do this from the beginning. If he does, he is probably trying to impress his analyst.

Free association is not only a discipline; it also represents a transgression. It transgresses the normal rules of conversation and in this sense gives a feeling of great freedom—to which Freud responded that the organizing principle of these associations is some other Law, the Law of the unconscious. Thus, as Lacan pointed out often, the associations are not free at all; they are strictly determined by Laws we ignore. In being a transgression of rules that are the stuff of normal human intercourse, this kind of speech produces an experience that makes the subject feel godlike. To have the privilege to say anything you like to someone else is not within the realm of possible experiences as lived by mortals. This aspect of psychoanalytic experience is extraordinarily appealing, and once people have gotten a taste of it it is extremely difficult to give up. It is certainly one of the important reasons why people choose to do psychoanalysis.

The analyst's encouragement to verbal incontinence permits the analysand to get away with saying things that he would never say normally. The analysand is requested to be impolite and uncivil, not to mince his words, especially as concerns his interlocutor. Courtesy and the amenities of normal communication are out of place here, as are considerations for the feelings of the listener. Whereas normal conversation attempts to gain some sense of mutual understanding leading to communication, psychoanalysis tries precisely to break down communication and whatever understanding the analysand had already arrived at. Free association dispenses with the logical connectives of neurotic discourse and attempts to discover another logic. For Lacan this new construction was something that emerged during the course of the analysis; it was rare that he himself made connections or constructions. Basically he waited for the patient to be able to connect things up for himself. And since during the course of analysis these connections were usually those of the neurosis, Lacan would content himself with signifying that such an interpretation was not right. We will see in a later chapter how Lacan worked; suffice it to say here that generally he let things slide as long as he could. He did not conceptualize his role as that of the interpreter, offering meanings for each dream and symptom. The tremendous intelligence we read in his writings was not something that he bandied about very often in sessions. The burden of interpreting as a regular, even a daily activity passed into the hands of the analysand. And as long as this activity was proceeding, which meant that the patient was offering different interpretations, Lacan let things move along at their own pace. His interpretations were limited to those occasions where the patient reached a point of certainty and conviction that caused the dialogue to stop.

Lacan as an analyst was not trying to establish any sort of communication with his patients; nor did he think it a good idea that they understand each other. Like most analysts he encouraged free association but did not listen to it as if it were the ranting of someone involved in a gratuitous sort of self-indulgence. Lacan, like most analysts, listened to something other than what was said; he listened as if the remarks that were about him were really addressed to someone else and as if the remarks of the analysand that were supposed to be about himself were really about an other. This he did without saying very much. By acting much of the time as if he were a creature from another planet, even another galaxy, Lacan gave the impression that he was hearing something other than what you were saying. He never put himself on the same wavelength as his analysand, but remained always at cross purposes. He never tried to find areas of agreement and accord, but scrupulously maintained a fruitful, well-tuned discord.

How much the analyst interprets depends largely on how much uncertainty he can tolerate. Lacan taught that you should never be too quick to fill in the blanks and to make sense of what you are hearing. He had confidence that with time the analysand would say what sense things had for him. One of the few things you can be sure of here is that, once that meaning is articulated, the analyst knows that it is the wrong one.

Analysis affords the opportunity for someone to say all the things he has never been able to say, to say them freely and without fear of punishment. It also permits him to hear things that he has never heard spoken to him. Not only does this procedure refuse to give the analysand recourse to a sense of guilt for what he is saying; it also dispenses with any consideration for his sense of Self. Now this differs from the view of most people these days, so the concept of Self will have to be elaborated.

Consider the idea of normal communication or conversation. There are a certain number of preconditions without which this cannot take place: civility and a reasonable balance between speaking and listening. When someone in a normal conversation addresses you, you are basically required to respond. You can't act as if the question were addressed to someone else. Also, one attempts in conversation to be coherent and to make some sort of rational sense. Finally, each speaker is expected to mean what he says, if not also to say what he means.

The speaker in a normal conversation is defined as identical to himself; he is thus taken to have a Self that he either expresses or presents. The Self does not talk about one thing to talk about another. Nor does it address one person to address another. Thus the speaking Self is the Self that is speaking, what it says is what it says, what it means is what it means, and the person to whom it addresses itself is the person to whom it addresses itself. The Self in other words is a principle of identity applied to a human subject. There can be no normal conversation where I as Self tell you as listener that the rain will make the flowers grow and where this means ultimately that there is an unconscious desire in me to perform an obscene act with your sister. And not only is this excluded from normal conversation, but normal conversation is based on this exclusion. In passing, note that this eventuality is also excluded from linguistics.

The normal conversation is an ideal. Thus when Chomsky talks of normal language usage, he posits an ideal speaker and ideal listener to engage in the hypothetical conversation that is the foundation of linguistic analysis. We would certainly admit that such conversations exist, though they require a degree of complicity between the participants. Such a practice provides a needed buffer between people; it keeps things running smoothly and permits life to go on. Eliminate the rules for normal conversation and people will become very aggressive; they will begin to tear each other apart. Obviously the terms of the kind of conversation that takes place in psychoanalysis should not generally and unreservedly be applied to everyday life. Human existence is not a therapeutic encounter.

The aspects of human existence revealed in psychoanalysis are truths that linguistics, with its passion for knowledge, cannot recognize. People may gain a sense of being alive by expressing a Self and by being reassured that what they are saying is being understood by the other, but they do not gain any sense of existence from it. They will suffer from this feeling of not existing.

As far as psychoanalysis is concerned, nothing within its purview should fall within the domain of the normal conversation. There is a fine example of this in a book entitled *The Basic Fault* by Michael Balint. Balint recounts how during an analytic session he tried to explain something to an analysand. The analysand did not understand, so Balint thought that perhaps he was not being clear enough. He restated the idea in more comprehensible language. The patient seemed to understand less than he had understood before, and repeated efforts at clarification produced even greater confusion.

This tells us that there is, within even the most innocent

remarks, an element of equivocation and that a person doing a psychoanalysis is not interested in having normal conversations with his analyst. In the transference the analyst is taken to be one who knows the truth of his patient's desire but who will never state that truth. The analysand will come to see that his analyst can only tell him this through riddles and enigmas. Thus he seeks from his analyst indications about his own desire, and he will think that every gesture, verbal or otherwise, is fraught with hidden meanings.

Having discovered this, Lacan advised analysts to say as much as possible of what they have to say through other than verbal means. Certainly they should avoid offering explanations and meanings. Qualities of flamboyance and demonstrativeness, of theatricality, are all to the better for the analyst, especially since they show a lack of inhibition on his part. The idea that the analyst is a blank screen on which the patient projects his fantasies is interesting but not entirely accurate. It does not mean that the analyst ought always to have a blank expression on his face. When the analyst gesticulates, when he moves around the room, when he alternates between being very kind and supportive and being uninterested and withdrawn, or even when he becomes an embodiment of the superego—as Lacan did on occasion—these are roles that an analyst may play as a character cast in a role that is not his. He suffers and he waits, sometimes patiently and sometimes with great impatience, for a word from the analysand that will deliver him from this plight.

The view from the transference would have it that everything the analyst does and says is meaningful. The analysand seeks signs—of love or hate or indifference. The role of the analyst is to point him beyond signs. One way Lacan did this was to adopt a facial expression that some might characterize as blank, but I saw it as best resembling a death mask. Faced with this representation of death, of a void, the analysand says whatever comes to mind without thinking of whether it is appropriate or not. His intention is to bring the mask back to life, to make it react and break its silence. The analysand tries to pin the analyst down into a human role, and this always fails. The process may be conceptualized as projecting on a blank screen; but what I am saying is that the cinematic metaphor is slightly off the mark. Something else is happening that could account for the same phenomena, and this something else, for the analysand, is a matter of life and death.

The analysand does not see himself in the death mask; he sees a representation of Otherness. I will offer some examples of Lacan's technique to make this unambiguous. One of his more interesting and exasperating gestures was arranging piles of banknotes on his desk, to sort and count them. You might think that this is the image of the miser counting his money. And within the transference an appropriate interpretation from the analysand would have been that the analyst only loves money and thus only receives his patients because they pay him. This interpretation is probably recognizable to anyone who has had some experience with analysis.

Yet is that what Lacan was saying with this gesture? The other way of reading it is to see that the analyst who signifies that he has a lot of money, as was Lacan's case, is also signifying to his patient that he is *not* doing it for money. In terms of desire, someone who has a lot of money is obviously not wanting for money, his desire is not countable in hundred-franc notes. The true question, Lacan was saying, is not who he loves or does not love, but what he desires. What does he, as analyst cast in the role of the grand Other, desire? This is the question the gesture poses, and the analysand does not want to hear it. The development of the analysis leads from the recognition that the analyst wants something to the analysand's telling him what he, the analyst, wants. Once the analysand articulates things in these terms, then the analyst interprets to signify that he wants—but that what he wants is not that.

Why in this case did Lacan make a gesture rather than offering an interpretation? The reason, as I understand it, is that money, however interesting a topic it may be for an analysand, is not what is really in question. It is one of any number of possible stumbling blocks on the path to posing the question of desire. The analysand should arrive at the point of stating what he wants or, better, what he thinks he wants. Then the analyst interprets; in his way he signifies the fact that what the analysand thinks the analyst wants is not one thing or another. The gesture as a way of saying something seems to be bound to the function of negation, not of denegation. The analyst is not denying anything with this gesture; he is simply pointing to where he is not, thus to where the analysand is casting him.

Another example is anecdotal and extra-analytic. It shows what manner of man Lacan was and how he reacted to particular situations. It will also show how Lacan won his reputation for being ill-mannered and somewhat daft. During the mid-seventies Lacan decided that he wanted to meet the film director Roman Polanski, and he asked a friend who knew Polanski to arrange a meeting. The friend invited the director and Lacan to have dinner in an elegant Paris restaurant. Lacan and his friend arrived at the restaurant first and were engaged in what I understand to have been normal conversation. Then Polanski arrived, sweeping across the restaurant with the kind of swagger that told everyone who he was. Notorious for his amorous exploits, he was accompanied by a ravishing young woman. Lacan observed this scene, was introduced to Polanski, and then emitted a loud, pronounced, and resonant sigh, the kind that would have been difficult to ignore five tables away. The director was somewhat taken aback by the gesture. Lacan sighed again, and again, and again. One might say that this is a wonderful way to greet an exhibitionist. At the least it shows why Lacan was said to have terrible public manners.

Strictly speaking, what Lacan was doing was beyond table manners. He was saying something that is not too difficult to understand. Seeing the demeanor, the bearing, the presentation of self affected by Polanski, Lacan responded: Who do you take me for, one of your groupies? He did not say this; he just sighed. Polanski, I gather, was not at all amused by the scene, especially insofar as Lacan had managed to up-stage him. The director placed himself in the camp of a not inconsiderable number of people who think when they hear such stories that Lacan was out of his mind.

I would only want to say here that such gesturing (as opposed to posturing) requires great discipline. It requires such discipline if it is to make sense within the social context in which it is offered. That it makes sense does not mean that the person to whom it is directed will grasp that sense. Once Lacan had stolen the scene or even the thunder of the famous director, it was for him to steal it back, if he dared to. Usually it is easier to denounce the Other as a madman. As for Lacan's contribution to the scene, I am saying that it would have been easier for him simply to sit by and make small talk, to spend the evening in a convivial, if empty, chat. It is easier to get along with people, to massage their egos in return for their massaging yours. This would have been normal and natural and pleasing to all involved. As I have said, this was not Lacan's way.

We can take this further by responding to a question I have often heard. Was Lacan conscious of what he was doing in scenes like the ones I have recounted? Could he have done otherwise? Were these acts thought out in advance? There clearly had to be a choice made by Lacan at some time or other to follow the path he followed. This judgment at its best would have been the consquence of a theoretical elaboration, a weighing of the effects produced, a decision that an act of speech produces an effect in the listener but does not communicate information about the state of one's feelings or the state of the world. Once this judgment was made, the rest followed, I would say, of its own desire. It would be too much to say that Lacan did not know what he was doing, that he was acting from intuition or even instinct. If I said this I would be saying that he was indulging himself or exercising some sort of antisocial tendencies. But the important point I want to make about these kinds of gestures is that they are precisely timed and placed in relation to what is offered; they are not gratuitous or senseless. They speak to the interlocutor whether he likes it or not, and they produce an effect. After the fact the scene, taken as a text, can be plumbed to find out what was going on, but I doubt that Lacan, when he emitted his first loud sigh, was thinking the kinds of things we can say when analyzing the event as a closed dialogue. Which is another way of saying that what happens during a psychoanalysis is grasped most truly when the analysis is over.

This returns us to the question that opened this chapter and that I will restate with a slightly different emphasis: What leads a subject to undertake psychoanalysis? Now this is precisely the question that the analysis is intended to resolve, and perhaps it is the only question it can address with any pertinence. Ultimately, the analysand's knowledge of the series of events that led him to the analyst's doorstep is not acquired until the end of the analysis.

The beginning of any psychoanalytic treatment engages a specific demand or question. The prospective analysand asks to be accepted into analysis, and he asks in addition that this analysis provide him with a cure or else with professional training. In Paris the demand to become a psychoanalyst was the question around which training analysis revolved, and it had to be addressed to the person you had chosen to be your analyst. In my case this is what I asked Lacan.

How did he handle it? The question was elaborated and

articulated throughout the development of the transference. It was posed specifically at certain crucial or crisis points in its unfolding. Periodically, the flow of associations and new material would grind to a halt, and this question of becoming a psychoanalyst would rear its head, like the Hydra confronting Hercules.

Lacan's response was to signify in one way or another that this was not the question, that if I thought I was there to become a psychoanalyst I was sorely mistaken. This was always a soul-rattling experience. Before you jump to a conclusion, I will say that he did not mean that I was there to be cured. In other psychoanalytic treatments, as I have suggested above, it is a mistake to take the demand for a cure at face value, as much of a mistake as it is to take the demand to be a psychoanalyst in that way. Lacan meant, as I discovered much later, that the constellation of factors that led me to psychoanalysis at a particular time, in a particular place, and with a particular analyst had nothing to do with the decision to become a psychoanalyst. Nor did it have anything to do with my aptitude for the profession, my abilities as an analyst, and so on. The question of why I decided to do a psychoanalysis was only answered by reference to the structure of my unconscious as it was played out in my personal history. Lacan made it clear, mostly in offhand remarks, the kind that do not appear to be of great importance, that this was what I should try to find out about. The question of being a psychoanalyst, as he said, can wait.

Why then were his interpretations directed almost entirely to aspects of the transference question? Perhaps for the same reason that Socrates said that he knew nothing except what concerned Eros. Lacan responded to questions that were directed to him and that concerned him directly, questions in which he was implicated and in which he had permitted himself to be implicated by accepting me into analysis. That was what he had to answer for, not my personal history.

7

THE DOOR TO THE BUILDING HOUSING LACAN'S OFFICE
was like other entrances to other French buildings. A very
large double door opened into a courtyard. Within that door
a smaller opening was cut to permit visitors to pass. The
smaller door was always locked but opened easily when you
pushed a small button on the right. With a brief buzz the
lock unlatched with a click to permit your passaage. It was as
if the French had spent centuries preparing for the arrival of
Freudian symbolism.

To reach Lacan's office you walked to the end of the
courtyard until you found a door on the right. Through that
and up a flight of stairs to a third door, a second buzzer;
there was no sign to indicate who was within. This door
was invariably opened by Lacan's secretary, Gloria, who
escorted you into the waiting room. One does not need too
much imagination to guess at the number of psychoanalytic
fantasies in which Gloria played a part. Certainly her assis-
tance was of major importance for Lacan. She worked with
him tirelessly for over thirty years, which ought to qualify
her for sainthood.

In 1973 the office and waiting room had an air of shab-
biness. They had not been painted for some time and there

were cobwebs everywhere. The carpeting was worn through in places, sign of the enormous traffic it had borne as well as of Lacan's inattention to his professional surroundings. The place was an island in time; I had the impression that aside from the traces of the passage of generations of analysands it had not changed in decades. During one summer while I was there Lacan finally had the place repainted and recarpeted, no doubt against his better judgment.

The waiting room was small, with just enough room for a loveseat and two easy chairs. Over the fireplace hung a signed portrait of St. Joseph, a souvenir portrait as it appeared to be. Was he the patron saint of Lacan's analysands? The table on one side of the loveseat contained within its surface postcardlike pictures of Rome, and on the other side was a magazine rack always filled with the latest issues of the French art magazine *l'Oeil*. Resting on the table was a piece of wood, which could have been driftwood or a sculpture, shaped precisely like an oversized phallus, the kind you would expect to find in a scene from de Sade. At other times this piece of wood resembled the trunk of an elephant raised as it would be were the elephant to talk.

The reference to de Sade is not entirely gratuitous. Lacan did at one time have a boxer dog that he named Justine. He told his seminar audience once that the dog could talk to him and even understood what he was saying to her. What made Justine different from people, he averred, was that she never took him for someone else.

Between the waiting room and Lacan's office was an unused room, containing a desk, desk chair, and a wall of bookcases. Beyond it to the right was a second waiting room, somewhat larger than the first, with several chairs and two walls of bookcases. This room was there to be called into service by the crush of people arriving at peak hours, between six and eight in the evening.

On the left and beyond the unused room was Lacan's office. The office itself was rather small, perhaps nine feet by fourteen, with the couch against one wall and Lacan's desk facing another. The walls were covered with drawings and some paintings, and there was one rather large African sculpture next to the desk. There were no bookcases, and the only other pieces of furniture were the leather chair behind the couch and a small easy chair at the other end of the room. Lacan was an important art and book collector, a man who by all reports lived in great luxury. None of this was evident in his office. Unless my insufficient knowledge of art prevented me from appreciating the quality of the work in view, there was nothing to distinguish Lacan's office from that of other psychoanalysts, nothing to suggest the enormous stature Lacan claimed for his work, nothing, in other words, to distract you from your encounter with Lacan.

Freud said that he wanted to prop his patients up with pillows so that, when they were lying on the couch, they would be almost sitting up. Lacan had patients lie flat on the couch with only a small pillow to raise the head. But the atmosphere was warm and comfortable, and for the first few interviews, the preliminary interviews, Lacan was a very gracious host. Always impeccably dressed, wearing a suit or sports jacket over a collarless shirt, tieless, his hand invariable holding a twisted cigar, Lacan was a man of medium height whose head seemed too large for his body, "hydrocéphale," as he said. His facial expression drew your immediate attention. He was convivial, friendly, acting to put his guest at his ease, not a very easy task. As a listener he was patient and attentive, exhibiting what seemed to be total concentration through an air of puzzlement. His look was fixed on his interlocutor as if to ask: Who are you and where did you come from? Since these interviews tended to take place in the early or middle afternoon, there was time to linger in conversation, even time on one occasion to drink a glass of Jack Daniels. Lacan pronounced it the best thing he had found in America.

This atmosphere was not to last very long. The beginning of the analysis proper was signaled by a gesture that made Lacan infamous in the world of psychoanalysis: the short session. The first one is doubtless the most memorable. You arrive for your session, let us say, in a fairly good mood, filled with things to say, about your past, your present, your fantasies, your dreams, whatever. The analysand has a lot to say because even the preliminary interviews have started to produce an effect: all sorts of things have come bubbling to the surface and nothing gives more satisfaction than to recount them to the friendly analyst. So you begin the session with some introductory remarks and pass to the subject you want to elaborate, to analyze, to ponder, to understand. You want the analyst to hear this because it is *really* important. But no sooner have you broached the topic, no sooner have the words identifying it passed through your lips, than Lacan all of a sudden rises from his chair and pronounces the session to be over, finished, done with. And he did this unceremoniously with a total lack of the good manners to which one is accustomed. When it's over it's over, no appeal, no going back, no revising or reconsidering. Whatever remained to be said would have to wait. The ending of the session, unexpected and unwanted, was like a rude awakening, like being torn out of a dream by a loud alarm. (One person likened it to *coitus interruptus.*)

Short sessions usually lasted only a few minutes. Their time was the time of a dream, the few minutes of sleep eked out before the inevitable awakening to the real. For the noise that draws us out of sleep is real; Lacan called it an exemplary instance of the real. He said that most people were something like somnambulists and that his role was to awaken them. In what was probably his last interview, published in the magazine *l'Ane*, he declared that the desire of death was not sleep or the dream, but the awakening. You awaken to desire and that desire is death—who would not want to remain asleep, if only for a few minutes?

The gesture of breaking the session, of cutting if off, was a way of telling people to put things to the side, to move forward, not to get stuck or fascinated by the aesthetics of the dream. As Augustine said in the *Confessions*: "And even thus is our speech accomplished by signs emitting a sound; but this, again, is not perfected unless one word pass away when it has sounded its part, in order that another may succeed it."

There was something of the horror of death in the short sessions, in these psychoanalytic sessions whose time could not be known in advance, whose time was not counted by the ticks of a clock. There were no magic numbers with Lacan, no fifty-minute hour, no five o'clock patient, at times not even a fixed number of sessions in a week. Eventually a degree of regularity was established, but Lacan never wanted things to be too precise; near the end of my analysis he said that I should come to my sessions at whatever hour I wanted.

So the analysand found himself thrown into reality, ejected into the world without so much as a fare-thee-well. I have introduced this subject with the desire of death because looking back this is the only way it makes sense to me. This was certainly not the way I lived the experience. On the contrary, I felt myself thrown into the transference and tried to understand what was happening, to mitigate the harshness of Lacan's desire, to seduce him into granting more time, to explain away what seemed to be the function of some unpredictable destiny, to assert the province of the ego over this thing that defied mastery, which was so little apt to be drawn into the sphere of consciousness that the sphere itself could only break under the strain.

The combined pressure of the shortness of the sessions and the unpredictability of their stops creates a condition that greatly enhances one's tendencies to free-associate.

When things come to mind they are spoken almost immediately, with spontaneity, for there is no time to mull them over, to find the nicest formulation. The analysand is encouraged, rather unsubtly, to get to the point, not to procrastinate or beat around the bush or even to prepare the analyst to hear disagreeable comments. Almost by definition the ego can never be the master of the short session.

This ego, however, does not just roll over and play dead. It asserts itself with a vengeance, not only in trying to control the situation but in offering interpretations of the analyst's bizarre behavior, attempting to situate it within the stages of psychosexual development. The stages of psychosexual development retain their pertinence in this practice and it is the analysand who tries, often with great perseverance, to maintain their explanatory function. This mode of interpretation is eventually revealed to be the system that holds the neurosis in place. If the analyst believes that bringing it into consciousness is salutary, he is providing a seal of approval for the neurotic condition. This does produce some changes in the attitude of the neurotic toward his neurosis, but it does not alter the structure in any fundamental way. This is why I introduced the short session under the heading of the death drive.

From this point of view there is no answer to the question that is often asked: How does the analyst know when the session is over? Certainly he does know, and he knows as a function of what he has heard. And what he has heard is not at all the same thing as what the analysand thinks he has said. The stops seem to be arbitrary, but that is because analysand and analyst are not on the same wavelength; they are not listening to the same thing. Whereas the analysand thinks that his ego is declaring its intentions to love or to hate or even to ignore, the analyst hears the discourse of the Other, the unconscious that slides through the gaps in intentionality. He wants the patient to hear it also. And after the analysand gets beyond such questions as why is he doing this to me?—after he gives up on trying to assert his control of the situation—he will hear his own unconscious and let it into his discourse.

Another question about the short sessions is how can anyone free-associate within such constraints. If one assumes that relaxation is conducive to free association, that a certain amount of time is required for the patient at least to settle in on the couch, then clearly Lacan's way of conducting sessions was not conducive to free association. Lacan kept people off balance, in a state of uncertainty as to what each session would bring. He doubtless felt that too much relaxation would only permit the ego's censorship to reassert itself. Certainly, it is possible for an analysand to go through the motions of talking freely, consciously erasing all connectives from his discourse, and not to free-associate at all. Are we that sure that we know what free association is all about?

Free associating is letting your mind wander, letting thoughts come to you without thinking or reflecting on each one as it comes. Once a thought makes itself known, it is put to the side to open a space in which a new thought can emerge. The question of why A leads to D instead of B is not asked; the associations emerge disconnected in a series or chain. This process is not like what we usually think of as letting one's mind wander. It is not daydreaming or elaborating fantasies. Each thought in free association is a discrete unit, counted as one, and no effort is made to form these thoughts into a whole or a unity that would have coherence and consistency. The presupposition, drawn from experience, beginning with Freud's, is that the last element in the series or chain will link the others in a way that could not have been grasped before this last element emerges. This is another way of saying that we do not know the meaning of a sentence until the final term is pronounced and until the punctuation is placed. At this point the questions that had necessarily been left suspended in the process of associating reassert themselves and find a response that could only have been guessed at beforehand. The assumption is that this method of proceeding provides a more direct access to the materials in the unconscious than does any conscious reflection. But, again, how do we know that a patient is truly free-associating? Is it possible, say, for an analysand to produce associations in a session that are not determined by the unconscious but that are simply the products of conscious reflection, where the associations have simply been chosen from previous conscious reflection? And how can we know that this process is not taking place in analysis as a function of the analysand's wish to be a good patient, to please the analyst?

Free association is not a normal way of thinking. Left to their own devices people do not free-associate; they keep their thoughts under the strict control of the ego, of the way the ego would like to see itself or of what it would like to think. Free association takes place under some duress. The process has to be motivated if it is to reach its term; comfort and relaxation cannot be part of the motivation. The reason for this is that in the series of associations it is always possible at one point or another to think that you have reached the end, the terminus, and that for the most part these points are points of resistance.

This brief look at the principle of free association will help to clarify what Lacan was doing with the short sessions. Most analysts have felt that the process of free association takes place *within* the analytic session, and this happened on occasion even with Lacan. What Lacan added was a free association that took place between sessions, in both senses of the word *between*. I said that each association is a discrete unit and that the associations are linked together as a series or chain. With short sessions each session was one association, and the series of associations corresponded to the series of sessions. The cutoff point said that the association just offered should not be lingered over but put aside to clear the mind to receive the next association. Thus it would happen that, as soon as I walked out of Lacan's office, a new thought would spring to mind, and this thought, or a series of associations it had elicited, became the subject of the next session. Lacan did not tell you to free-associate, did not cajole or convince you of the worthiness of this procedure. What he did do was to construct the sessions so that that was what you were obliged to do.

Sessions with Lacan were almost always open-ended; they always left something more to be said. Lacan never tried to tie things up, to make them come together into a unifying statement of a meaning. This the patient did for himself and he did it around the transference, around the idea that he had formed of the analyst and of the analytic relationship. Lacan was critical of therapists who tried to treat one question per session, to attempt to resolve it so as to move on to the next question. The associations in a series are not resolutions representing a unity, but they are strictly countable units. Lacan emphasized the difference between the countable one and the unifying one, and his practice is understood best in these terms.

I said that there were no magic numbers with Lacan's sessions, no fifty-minute hour and such. Yet each session counted as one, as a unit, almost at times as a trait representing difference. And it did not matter how long the session lasted or did not last; it was still one session and was charged or counted as one. When I say that the sessions could become pure traits representing difference, I mean that the session represented a break in the continuity of everyday life, a break in the humdrum quality of the lives that most poeple lead. And certainly Lacan's sessions were that; his way of timing things was not at all the same as the rest of life, where the clock most often is master.

Another point should be emphasized here. Lacan's short session was the technique that was most contested by those who knew about it. Lacan did not encourage others to follow exactly the same technique, and few other Parisian analysts, even Lacanians, had sessions as short as his. The principles involved in short sessions are also operative in longer sessions. This means that the most relevant associations are not likely to be the ones produced within the session but the ones produced between the sessions. It is very rare for an analysand to make an important discovery while free-associating in session; discoveries made this way are generally suspect.

There is more to psychoanalysis than free association. Some analysts believe that the process of psychoanalysis concerns the forming of synthetic ideas that encompass the meaning of a neurosis. In this way the ego gains mastery over id impulses. There have even been analysts who have proposed that psychoanalysis is a misnomer, and that the procedure should be called psychosynthesis. This search for unity, to find some sort of unification, obviously ran counter to Lacan's theory and practice. The purpose of the short session was to focus on a particular point, or a series of points, which was structuring for the rest. The sessions did not encourage synthetic statements but rather something that can be called a verbal gesture, a short concise statement of where one is at any particular moment. This kind of statement, which tended toward the aphoristic, is not a function of the ego but rather a function of the intellect, the mind.

People in analysis often yield up a mass of verbiage whose purpose is to confuse the issue and to cloud over the question. Lacan must have felt that talking too much often was used as a resistance to avoiding the issues. Something about the freedom to say anything that comes to mind is simply too satisfying for the analysand, and this intense satisfaction, often experienced as an erotic satisfaction, is a barrier to desire.

Through the experience of short sessions the analysand learns first to get right to the point and second to say as much as possible quickly. This requires a command of language, an access to the possibilities that language offers that is beyond what people ordinarily make use of. To learn to deploy language to say exactly what you want to say without wasting words is a discipline that requires training. The short session offers the opportunity for a new dialogue between the subject and his language. I am not talking about something that requires an exceptionally high IQ. Among the instances of the mobilization of intellect must be counted the uses of wit and jokes. These are hardly limited to those who have had a high level of formal education.

Lacan's short sessions were not always a cause célèbre. I want here to examine the role they played within the psychoanalytic groups in Paris and how they tampered with a sacred ritual. When Lacan started doing short sessions, he presented the technique as an experiment before his psychoanalytic society. The society considered the practice worthy of discussion in the late 1940s or early '50s. Lacan then presented some of the candidates who had been trained with this technique so that the society could judge the effectiveness of the training analyses. In most if not all cases the relevant committee judged that the technique was analytically competent and effective. I mention this point to underscore the fact that Lacan did not introduce short sessions as a gesture of defiance or as a transgression of the rules of his psychoanalytic society. Also the first judgment of his practice, rendered before Lacan had become notorious, was interested and skeptical.

The issue came into prominence in the split of the Paris society that took place in 1952. Lacan as a leader of the dissidents was accused at that time of a number of things, of having resigned from the society defiantly, of corrupting the youth of Paris, and so on. Eventually, the rancor against the dissidents crystallized around the issue of the short sessions. Later, in the early sixties, when the International Psychoanalytic Association pronounced Lacan incompetent to teach and train candidates, it picked up on the issue of the short session and even did a study concluding that it was a bad practice. The IPA committee decided that the short session increased the dependence of the analysand on the analyst and therefore prolonged the length of the analysis unduly. The practice was also considered to be directive and manipulative, lacking the kind of objectivity and scientificity inherent in sessions run by the clock.

It is not untrue that analysis with Lacan often lasted many many years. Perhaps the average was something like seven to nine years for a training analysis; some lasted longer and others less. But this duration for analytic treatment was not peculiar to Lacan. Analyses that last a very long time are commonplace in parts of the world where Lacan has had no influence. This probably has to do with the refinement that analytic technique has undergone since the time of Freud. Certainly Freud's analyses lasted a much shorter length of time.

That the short session produces in the analysand something like an infantile dependence is basically false. In the first place the short sessions did not produce real regressions (a friend in analysis in England told me that he had regressed to the oral phase and therefore had given up eating solid foods). Lacan did not want people to act like three-year-olds, and his analysands generally did not. The use of regression for Lacan was limited to what he called rememoration, which concerned remembering past experiences not as they were lived the first time but in terms of the important signifying elements that remained from them in the unconscious.

It is true that people in analysis with Lacan have tended to exhibit more passions with less control than those in analysis with analysts of the IPA. This is somewhat difficult to demonstrate, but note that the problem of the inability to love, posed by Otto Kernberg and others in the United States, never attracted much attention in France. The reason was not so much a theoretical divergence as the fact that love is more important in French life than it is in the United States or England. I will simply note the point made earlier, that

Lacan does merit some criticism for overzealously stoking passions, but making this criticism does not require that we reject Lacan's theory *in toto* or that we close our eyes to the issues and questions he raised with the short session.

One observation about the bitter debate over short sessions imposes itself at this point. Lacan was criticized so vehemently for one basic reason: the issue was an easy one to grasp and thus gave a reason to condemn Lacan. Having condemned him on this one question, people could blithely proceed to ignore everything else that he had to say about psychoanalysis. The short session became a rallying cry, a threat to the integrity of a sacred ritual, and this permitted the establishment of a consensus opposed to Lacan. Members of the group of psychoanalysts had only to know that Lacan practiced short sessions to formulate an opinion about his theoretical work. Holding to this belief was requisite for members in good standing of the group.

Lacan's theoretical work, representing a challenge to the predominant consensus that had formed around the theory of ego psychology, was relegated to the realm of the unspeakable. In 1952 Lacan published a paper entitled "Reflections on the Ego" in the *International Journal of Psychoanalysis*. The next Lacan text to be published in a journal run by members of the IPA was a paper on the case of the Rat Man, published in the *Psychoanalytic Quarterly* in 1979. The condemnation of Lacan by the International was effective. And it was effective primarily on the ground of the short session because this was the only thing about Lacan that most analysts knew. Unfortunately, or fortunately, Lacan was a ghost who refused to play dead.

Lacan had managed to put into question the psychoanalytic session itself, the session as ritual. The difference between the fifty-minute hour and the short session is a difference between two concepts of time. On the one side time is fixed with precision; on the other, it is approximate and variable. More precisely, in the fifty-minute hour there is a guarantee that the session will have a particular duration, will take place in time, while the short session tends toward a point in time, an interval in which there is no time (as in "no time to speak"). The short session does not erase the duration of time, which is preserved in the time it takes to do an analysis, but the session itself becomes a break in the continuity of time; it marks time and thus structures it. Finally, in the normal psychoanalytic hour it is the clock that decides the ending of the session, which passes judgment in a purely arbitrary manner but, one might say, fairly, even-handedly. No matter who you are and what you are saying, the session, in principle, ends when fifty minutes have elapsed. In Lacan's short session the analyst adopts a role like that of a god who determines time, who decides the end of the session in a way that is not arbitrary and does not erase the subjectivity, what most would call the individuality, of the analysand. Rather it accentuates that subjectivity while at the same time making it appear that the analyst is arranging things for his own convenience. A Parisian analyst once tried to explain the short session by saying that Lacan was claustrophobic.

I am not asking the question of what time is. Rather I am pointing to the issue of whose time it is. When Lacan talked about why he invented the short session, he referred in particular to this question. He said that some analysands, knowing that they were guaranteed fifty minutes no matter what, used their sessions to discuss things that did not interest them in the least. If they had something important to say, they would wait for the last few minutes of the session to broach it. Lacan reasoned that such analysands were using the fifty-minute hour as a resistance, as an excuse to waste time—in particular, to waste the analyst's time, to make him wait for them. This is a neurotic form of abuse that finds a home in the fifty-minute hour. It is also called procrastination. The short session responds that the time being wasted is the analyst's and that he has some say in how he spends his time.

Some people may object here. Given that procrastination exists and that neurotic patients often bring it with them into their analysis, why wouldn't one try to analyze the procrastination, offering a sage interpretation instead of tampering with the time of the session? This alteration of the time of the session sounds like what Franz Alexander called a corrective emotional experience, and everyone knows that this idea has been discredited.

Alexander states in simple terms that, if an analysand is suffering from not having received enough love, then the analyst ought to show him love and affection. If the analysand grew up in an atmosphere where he was bathed in emotional effusions, the analyst should be withdrawn and controlled. And Alexander felt that alterations in time—especially in the frequency of sessions—were helpful in that context. Lacan's approach differed because he did not think that analysis should intervene in relation to emotional states; nor should it attempt to manipulate those states. Lacan sought an alteration of the relational structures that produced emotion. He felt that analysis should offer another structure, a structure that was not identical with that of everyday life. Thus the analytic situation, followed by most analysts, countenances free association, a form of verbal behavior that is unacceptable in other, more normal social situations. The short session is simply an extension of the principle that determines the analytic setting.

An interpretation of procrastination could be something like the following: You are making me wait because your mother always made you wait before eating. This may bring about a rise in conscious awareness, but there is no reason to believe that such a gain will necessarily produce a modification in the way you procrastinate. Now this is somewhat mysterious because it seems to contradict the theory. If we see it as putting the patient in a double bind, then perhaps it will be less mysterious. On the one hand the analyst offers an interpretation of a behavior pattern that has come to infest the sessions. Implicit in this interpretation is the idea that the patient ought to do otherwise. But at the same time the condition that encouraged the procrastination, provided a culture for it to grow in, the fifty-minute hour, remains inviolate. I hypothesize that Lacan thought things out in similar fashion when he decided that time was too important a factor in the cure to remain unquestioned.

Remember also that when the analyst requires the analysand to free-associate, he does not simply offer an interpretation of why the patient does not comply with this request. What he does and what he has always done is to provide conditions that encourage and facilitate this mode of expression. Thus the reclining position of the analysand, the place of the analyst behind him and out of his line of sight, the analyst's silence and his general refusal to engage in conversation or to reveal aspects of his own personality. All of these technical factors in the analytic situation sustain the offer to free-associate. If the analyst were to offer an interpretation and then sit facing the patient in a chair and engage in conversation with him about the weather, we can understand that his interpretation, however psychoanalytic it may be, will not produce much of an effect. And this is why, faced with analysands whose neurosis was intimately involved with procrastination, Lacan felt he had to introduce the short session and thereby another concept of time.

Procrastination gives every appearance of being an ethical concept. You find yourself faced with an unmistakable obligation to do something, you know that this is the act you should perform, that this act conforms perfectly with your desire, and yet you wait, you think, you procrastinate. Procrastination means not acting according to your desire; ultimately it produces guilt, not only for inaction but also for acting one way when your desire is elsewhere. In this, as in hasty actions, we say that your timing is off, your experience of time has stood in the way of your acting in accord with your desire.

Why delay things, and what are the things you wish to delay? In the seminar "Desire and Its Interpretation" (parts of which have recently appeared in *Ornicar?*) Lacan says that the obsessional neurotic wants to delay the encounter with death, to put off—indefinitely, if he can—this moment of truth. His reason is that he is not ready, but of course the obsessional is never ready; there is always some more preparing that must take place before he confronts his destiny.

Faced with death's desire the neurotic turns away, saying: Not now. This gesture derives from his interpretation of that desire; he feels that death wants his life, nothing more or less. And this life, whatever its worth, is something he wants to hold on to as long as possible. That death should be aiming for this life is what gives that life its value; this makes the obsessional feel somewhat alive.

The moment of truth, the encounter with death's desire, approaches through the counting of time. The succession of countable intervals leads in only one direction, and that is what the obsessional is not ready for. Thus he procrastinates, and the sense of this procrastination is to slow down the count, to create a duration, a flow of time in which there is no count, in which nothing counts. Except of course the obsessional himself who may create any number of rituals in which he is obliged to count, for example, to some magic number while he is in the process of washing his hands or face or hair. This gives him the assurance that he controls the count, that he knows it in advance, that he will not be caught unawares, and essentially that there is no other count but his, no count in the unconscious. To which Lacan replied by saying that the unconscious certainly counts, counts the number of sessions, the amount of money spent, the length of time the analysis has lasted, even attaching meanings to certain time periods or dates.

Note that if it should happen that the desire of death is not for the obsessional's life, then he certainly has a problem. Better, the fact that death's desire is not for life is what creates the problem. Like any other desire, death's desire is to be recognized and taken into account. In religious practice and rituals this is done through offerings, through sacrifice. To offer a part of himself to death's desire, this is too much to bear; better it were his life that death wants. The obsessional generally has a premonition that tells him which part of himself death wants to receive as an offering, and that is precisely the part the obsessional thinks is the key to life. As it happens with many religions, the obsessional neurotic thinks that his experience of sexual satisfaction should be properly directed toward the reproduction of life forms. Rather than think that this experience of *jouissance* is an experience of death, at least for the sexual organ that is involved, the obsessional would rather play dead, like an embalmed corpse. This is to trick death's desire, to avert its gaze from someone who is clearly not worth the trouble. The neurotic feels that were he to act this would betray him to death, not only showing a sign of life but also setting the count in motion. The intervals of time, being countable, require points or signposts, signifiers of difference, to move forward. And since he procrastinates to erase these signposts, the temporal expression that most clearly summarizes his subjective position, as Lacan said, is: Too late.

This is not the way things happen in hysteria. Freud said that hysterics suffer from reminiscences, from a past that has not been dealt with, from a mourning process that has not reached its term, from the unburied dead. The hysteric may try to forget the dead but the dead do not forget her. (The great majority of cases of hysteria are to be found in women—thus the feminine pronoun.) Not that the obsessional neurotic does not have some sort of relationship with the dead. His ritual in one sense is for their benefit. Faithful servant of death, the obsessional buries the dead and then reburies them, and does the same thing again and again and again. One has to be certain that they will stay buried, as if death had only one desire and that was the proper disposition of mortal remains. Not only does the obsessional not forget the dead, not repress them, but he is too solicitous of them, anxious about the satisfaction of death's desire. This is why his ultimate encounter will be with death itself; as much as he fears this encounter, he knows that this is the one that counts.

For the hysteric the dead remain alive, as living memories: sometimes as people who are remembered, who are grieved excessively—mourning and grief are not the same thing as ritual burial—as it happens in depression, but also as repressed memories that are converted into flesh, one might say, in what are called conversion symptoms. This is what happened in Breuer's case of Anna O., especially since her hysteria dated to the scene at her father's deathbed. The scene may or may not be repressed and forgotten, but the reminiscence remains alive in attacking some part of the body as a constant reminder of what was and is no longer. The hysteric's procrastination is an effort to keep the past alive, most especially in her body, considered or interpreted as fulfilling itself most truly in the reproduction of life. If the hysteric's question revolves around the meaning of femininity—in both male and female hysterics—the answer or interpretation she latches onto most often is that femininity is motherhood. As Moustapha Safouan said in his article "In Praise of Hysteria" (in my *Returning to Freud*) hysterics are remarkably well informed about every aspect of the experience of pregnancy. About their own sexuality hysterics are far less well informed.

Procrastination is a function of the ego. We have learned to think of the ego within the framework of a visual system of representation. For Lacan the ego is discovered by the infant as his mirror image. The ego reflects and observes, imparts an order to spatial representation. The narcissistic attachment to the ego, the promotion of its claims to sovereignty and strength and sanity, represents also a bias toward the life drives, toward Eros. Whether the ego engages itself in the effort to negotiate the moment of its own demise, thus to make this moment a triumph, illusory as it may be, or whether the ego functions to protract mourning, thus to retain the dead in life, it desires, as Freud said in *The Ego and the Id*, "to love and to be loved." Or, "to the ego, therefore, living means the same as being loved." How then could anyone set up his theory, as Lacan did, in opposition to the ego?

Freud says in the same paper that normally the ego permits us to give up lost love objects. It does this by delaying the moment when we are obliged to recognize our loss. Freud describes this in the following way: "When it happens that a person has to give up a sexual object, there quite often ensues an alteration of his ego which can only be described as a setting up of the object inside the ego, as it occurs in melancholia . . . It may be that by this introjection, which is a kind of regression to the mechanism of the oral phase, the ego makes it easier for the object to be given up or renders that process possible. It may be that this identification is the only condition under which the id can give up its objects. At any rate the process, especially in the early phases of development, is a very frequent one, and it makes it possible to suppose that the character of the ego is a precipitate of abandoned object-cathexes and that it contains the history of those object-choices" (Standard Edition, XIX, 29).

If the character of the ego always retains traces of lost objects, then we must say that these objects are never entirely relinquished. The ego becomes what the id wanted sexually. Comparing the process to melancholia does not give it the best credentials. The temporality engaged here certainly falls within the range of the concept of procrastination. Thus I give this process a somewhat more negative slant than Freud seems to have done. And I should also say that the identification of living with loving, however much it corresponds to what we would all like to think that life is all about, is highly debatable.

Procrastinating is not the same as deferring or delaying. Deferring an action assumes that when the time is right the action will be performed, that the subject who wants to sail a boat will defer his act until the wind is right. If the wind is right and he still does not sail, then he is procrastinating. The structure of procrastination is that the ego wishes to make desire into an ego function, wants to make desire its own. Once the lost object is taken into the ego, it becomes coextensive with the ego and the ego thinks that what the id desires is precisely the ego itself, not the trace of a lost object. The ego then thinks that it is loved and that being loved is what it desires, as Freud told us, but it goes one step further and declares that being loved is all that is wanted, that in being loved desire is satisfied, which successfully parries the desire of death. The ego does not interact with the desire of another and this is evident in the expressions from everyday language that use this term: egotistical, egoism, egomania. Now many of my colleagues would object here that these words do not use the same term as the psychoanalytic theory has defined. But often the meanings a term has acquired in ordinary language usage are more indicative than the meanings that are arbitrarily attributed to it in our technical jargon. If language, as Lacan says, is located in the Other, and if the meanings of words represent the desire of the Other, then is it not precisely an ego function to say that words mean what I want them to mean or, better, that the meaning of a word can be changed if enough of us get together and decide, reach a consensus, that it means something else? In the case in point here, we see a reversal within some branches of psychoanalytic theory of the value placed on the ego. The theory would have it that it is good to have a strong ego, that this ego is lovable and deserving of love, whereas for Lacan the ego is fundamentally paranoid. Living only for passion, for a love that would last forever, the ego, like the paranoiac, sees the Other's desire as a menace.

Lacan has been accused of reading Freud idiosyncratically. In *The Ego and the Id* Freud said: "We now see the ego in its strength and in its weaknesses. It is entrusted with important functions. By virtue of its relation to the perceptual system it gives mental processes an order in time and submits them to 'reality-testing.' By interposing the processes of thinking, it secures a postponement of motor discharge and controls access to motility"(XIX, 55). Lacan probably read this passage as saying that the longer the postponement, the stronger the ego. The question is: What counter-mechanism exists to stop the postponement, to precipitate an act? The problem is that this hypothetical counter-mechanism contradicts the mechanism that postpones. If the ego obeys the law of noncontradiction, and if this distinguishes it from the unconscious in which contradictory thoughts coexist, then the ego can only delay things. Left to its own devices, it makes that postponement into something pathological.

The point I want to make here is that it is only the intercession of the desire of the Other that precipitates action and breaks the cycle of delay. And I must add, so that there will be no misunderstanding, that it is not thought per se that is the culprit; it is rather the "I think," the belief that the ego is the center of thinking. Remember that in his paper on "The Unconscious" Freud situated thought in the unconscious and declared that what the ego perceives as thought is only a shadow or reflection of a thought process that is going on elsewhere. To echo Lacan (in "The Agency of the Letter in the Unconscious"), it is when I think I am thinking that I procrastinate. I must have time to think that I am thinking, to think that I am the conscious subject of my thoughts, and this is precisely what Lacan would not allow. The thoughts whose provenance is most clearly unconscious are those that come to me when I do not think to think. These are thoughts that surge forth; they are the stuff of free association, and they emerge in the gap created by the break in the time of the session. With Lacan's short sessions the analysand did not have time to get his bearings, to establish his sense of being in control of the situation, to get his thoughts in order.

Analysts object to this on the following grounds. They feel that Lacan, in refusing to make any alliances with the ego—and he was categorical on this point—in showing interest basically in what Freud called primary process material, had to provoke a state of psychic disintegration. Without a functioning ego, an ego that received some support and sustenance from the analyst, this primary process material would fly off into the ozone and would never be integrated.

To restate this in terms of Freud's idea of the ego's permitting the subject to accept the loss of a sexual object, performing something like an incomplete mourning rite—incomplete because the character of the ego is formed of the precipitates of abandoned object-choices—the question becomes: How can we deal with the dead without the mediating function of the ego? The answer becomes fairly obvious. We bury them, according to the rituals of our society, which is to say that we resituate them in a discourse. Personal grief exists in the frame of a discourse, and only the reference to discourse will prevent that grief from becoming chronic.

This is Lacan's response to the anxiety of those who would entrust the ego with the function of burying the dead, of dealing with loss. In Lacan's terms, we give the dead over to the symbolic order; their fate is not in the hands of anyone's ego. The case where the ego finds the justification for its work of mourning is precisely that in which someone had "died" but is not dead. Someone is dead-to-me, no longer loved or loving, but that someone, being dead-to, is not dead-too. When the experience of love is made out to be primary, the dominion of the ego is extended and death is reduced to a loss of love. The ego denies death by idealizing love and life; the dead remain alive in the strong ego, still loving and beloved. Thus the ego may recover from its loss by believing that, through death, love has been made eternal.

What Lacan was saying, though perhaps he did not say it just like this, was that the loss of love or the loss of what Freud called a sexual object is only negotiated through reference to the symbolic order. It is through the symbolic order and through the rituals it prescribes that the object is truly given up, truly buried. And if this person is not buried, metaphorically, which means forgotten, the subject will have no sense of loss or lack and will be alienated from a desire that can only be seen as a threat to the perfect harmony of the truest love.

Burying the past does not mean annihilating it. A living memory ought not to remain in the ego to captivate and fascinate, but this does not mean that nothing remains. From the point of view of the ego, a failure to remember does mean that nothing remains; thus the ego is the seat of nihilism. The image of the beloved is not the same as the trace of that person's passage. Someone who has been buried leaves a mark behind, a trace of his passage through our world. And that trace is inscribed indelibly in the unconscious—assuming that the object-choice and object-investment was made during early childhood. The investment of the image as it is reflected in the ego captures the subject's look so that the mark of the passage becomes unreadable. And this capture exists in what the ego would like to think of as a timeless present, an eternity in which the count of time has been suspended. Thus the ritualized imposition of the short session restores the count of time, subverts the ego in its procrastination, and permits the cipher of destiny to be read.

The emphasis on ego formation and development is common to contemporary theories of psychoanalysis and psychology. It is also seen in phenomena as diverse as what we call "the *me* decade," the idealization of youth and childhood as possessing some special and uncorrupted truth, the thorough lack of respect for the elderly, the failure to honor the dead. To the ego as autonomous entity is given the task of compensating for a failure at symbolization. The ego does not make this choice, but the choice is imposed upon it. The ego embraces it enthusiastically as if there were no other choice.

The best example that comes to mind is *Hamlet*. Kurt Eissler in *Discourse on Hamlet: A Psychoanalytic Study* argues that the development of the character of the protagonist of this play corresponds to the stages of ego development. So be it. That the greatest of procrastinators should represent the ego is perfectly consistent with what I have been saying. And nothing is more clear in the play than the fact that it is a failure to mourn the death of King Hamlet that creates the conditions in which the ego becomes predominant. What the play tells us is that the ego, even in so grand and poetic a character as Hamlet, is fundamentally inadequate to the task at hand; the ego cannot compensate for a failure at symbolization, for a breakdown in the social structure. Not only does the ghost return, but ultimately we must see the play as the triumph of the ghost of King Hamlet. The ghost becomes Death itself, and ultimately Death is the only one to sit down at table, to feast on the living, as the play tells us. Hamlet, for his part, is the major force in the arrangement of this repast. That he does finally carry out the ghost's command, that he kills his uncle, is not open to doubt. But when he does it, it is too late, his act no longer means anything, it no longer has its ethical edge. The murder of Claudius is an afterthought, which Hamlet, as Lacan said, can only accomplish when he is dying, when he will not have to bear responsibility for his act. Even more important is the fact that Hamlet acts when he learns that the wretched Claudius is responsible for Hamlet's impending death. Hamlet can avenge himself because he is an egoist to the end, especially at the end. With his dying breath he asks Horatio to tell *his* story. Perhaps his act is the sign of a mature and adult ego structure; if so, it is a powerful argument against anyone who would set up such a structure as a standard for ethical conduct. What Hamlet accomplishes, and this is perhaps his great achievement as a dramatic character, is to make himself lovable. A professor who taught me Shakespeare in college made the point that it is extremely puzzling that audiences love Hamlet so much: after all, he is a brutal murderer who shows little remorse in dispatching his victims.

Hamlet could rise to the occasion only when the clock was running out on him. He did what he knew he had to do only when the time was fixed. Thus ended his procrastination—but the act he performed was no longer the same act he would have committed had he done it at the right time. And in the meantime many other people died. To say that Hamlet shows the stages of ego development is accurate as a description; it does not address the ethical issue. Here Hamlet is clearly a failure—he cannot act on his desire, he can only perform the act he is obliged to perform when it is no longer his desire—and his success is to convince the audience that it is no failure at all, that we can still love him.

Lacan, then, refused to be a slave to the clock. He was not performing experiments during analytic sessions and never thought of his office as a laboratory. Some analysts have introduced this analogy to justify the fifty-minute hour, but if this is true, and if the analyst is a scientist, then the analysand is left to be the object of an experiment, material to be acted upon. Even if that were true, what scientist would refuse to shorten the time for an experiment, and what physician today would insist that the time of a consultation or even a surgical procedure is an absolute?

Lacan did not think that applying psychoanalytic theory to his practice was equivalent to following a tried and true recipe. He did not believe that less time would leave the dish undercooked, indigestible, or inedible. Nor did he think that the psychoanalytic session was like a religious ritual, which had to follow the prescribed form in order to be effective. It was not for him a learning experience, a classroom, in which the number of hours means exactly that, a time during which instruction is to be given in exchange for a payment. Lacan was evidently not bothered by the fact that a short session could never permit the patient to think things over, to enclose things within the net of his consciousness. For him psychoanalysis was the enemy of all that.

I have presented the short session in its starkest form, the form in which Lacan himself practiced it. I have chosen to present the strong case for it because nothing is to be gained by defensiveness. I should mention finally that Lacan was one of very few Lacanian analysts who practiced this technique in its most radical form, in the form where the time of the session became no time. Had I emphasized this, I would have made the practice into an idiosyncrasy, harmless or harmful as you will. And those who experienced these sessions did not feel that this was just another quirk of the Old Man. They would never have put up with it for so long in such great numbers if they had thought so. It is nonsense to say, as some anti-Lacanian Parisian analysts did, that Lacan's patients were mostly masochists.

Even if you believe that I am not the best judge of what was happening in my own analysis, my own judgments of Lacan's practice were refined through long discussions with many people who were or had been in analysis with him. These people were in different stages of their analyses, and over the years it was clear to the eye what the treatment was or was not doing for them. For the most part, what it was doing was positive.

Some might want to ask how Lacan got away with it. Certainly it was not his theoretical wizardry or his holding of positions of power in psychiatric institutions. He got away with it because he was an excellent clinician. This was his reputation, and it was one of the main reasons that so many psychiatrists and psychologists flocked to hear him explain how he did it. You can only go so far in trying to explain away Lacan by invoking phenomena of cults and followers. There is a bottom line in psychoanalysis, and it is quite simply the effectiveness of the treatment. On this psychiatrists and psychologists are not likely to be duped. I am not saying that Lacan never made mistakes or that every treatment he undertook turned out well. I would simply assert from my own experience and from that of many friends and acquaintances that the practice of the short session made a significant and substantial contribution to the success of Lacan's practice.

8

ONE IS TEMPTED TO OFFER A PSYCHOANALYTIC EXPLANA-
tion for Lacan. There was a time when I thought that the
key to Lacan's career lay in his relationship with his own analyst, Rudolph Loewenstein. Perhaps Lacan's analysis had
not been terminated properly, and he felt he had been abandoned when Loewenstein emigrated to the United States.
This would explain why Lacan was so preoccupied with the
question of the end of analysis, of the passage between the
place of the analysand and that of the analyst. Add to this
the fact that Loewenstein participated with Heinz Hart-
mann in the development of the theory of ego psychology
and one could also explain why Lacan felt that this theory
represented a betrayal of psychoanalysis, of Freud, of those
who had remained behind, of those who had returned to re-
build Europe after the war.

This hypothesis adds that Lacan undertook teaching in a
vain effort to find an analyst who would help him terminate
his analysis. And when the people he had trained turned
their backs on him, when they showed themselves to be inadequate, he turned on them with the same fury he had
shown toward those who had embraced the American way
of life and who seemed to have forgotten their European her-

itage. That psychoanalysis seemed to have left Europe in the lurch was intolerable to Lacan. There were in Europe and probably there still are a considerable number of people who blamed Woodrow Wilson for the advent of Adolph Hitler. When in doubt, blame the Americans.

This explanation is one I concocted one day in the heat of the transference; I did not hesitate to throw it at Lacan. He did not dismiss it out of hand; nor did he accept it with open arms. He was willing to accept some responsibility for the turmoil that swirled around him for the last thirty years of his life. And however much we believe that thoughts about one's analyst are the consequence of an overheated intellect, this does not necessarily make them false.

Lacan may have been a psychoanalyst like the others, but he was also a part of intellectual history, a figure who was larger than life and who represented for his students and followers something that could never be comprised by the idea that he was simply cultivating the psychoanalytic garden, reading, as it were, the Freudian text. Needless to say, when people began calling him a "phenomenon" and when some journalists declared in the *Nouvel observateur* that our age would be called the Age of Lacan, he greeted these statements with derision and contempt. This is not to say that Lacan was humble or modest in his own appraisal of his accomplishments. To have affected modesty would have been what the French call *con*, and no one ever accused Lacan of being *con*.

The era of conflict within his psychoanalytic world began after the war. It was not only the psychoanalysts who were at each other's throats; France itself was divided, and violently so, over the experience of the occupation and liberation. Denunciations for collaboration and betrayal were a part of the social and political fabric of the country.

Everybody knows or believes that the French are extremely xenophobic. At the same time, the French are intensely proud of their country and their culture. Men and women who have made important contributions to the society and culture are revered by the populace. It is difficult for a foreigner to understand the extent to which French pride was devastated by the Second World War. To appreciate this is also to appreciate the importance attached to any contributions that moved in the direction of the restoration of that pride. It was within this context that Lacan lived and worked. Lacan was French with a vengeance; he rarely if ever criticized his society, his culture, his civilization. Such a critique, an attack on the roots of the disaster of the war, could only be presented in circumlocutions. Lacan's work was not simply that of an everyday psychoanalyst; he rendered a service to his society that it would be hard to overestimate. If he did not do this through direct intervention in the political process, through condemnations of western civilization, one of the reasons was that he wanted to address questions that he must have felt could not be addressed directly. Rather than force people to confront things that they were incapable of confronting, he worked slowly and patiently on questions that people could study fruitfully. This is consistent with the work of psychoanalysis, where interpretation must be offered in terms of questions that the patient is ready to assume and resolve.

At the end of the war Europe was in ruins, physically, intellectually, spiritually. On top of the enormity of the human suffering there was the realization, articulated well by George Steiner in *Language and Silence*, that a civilization that had produced some of the world's greatest art, philosophy, literature, music, and science had also foisted on us one of the greatest abominations the world had known. The French experience of the war was obviously very different from the German. As far as culture is concerned, the German experience spoke clearly to all of those who had placed some faith in human intellect and human creativity. When Steiner points out that the guards at Auschwitz spent their leisure time reading Goethe or Rilke, or playing Bach and

Schubert, he adds that this poses a serious question about how we can continue to believe that anything is to be gained by the practice of the arts, to say nothing of philosophy. The country that gave us Bach, Goethe, and Kant also gave us Buchenwald, Dachau, and Treblinka. Perhaps there is a connection between the refinement of the human spirit and the wanton destruction of human life. As Steiner said, "it is at least conceivable that the focusing of consciousness on a written text ... diminishes the sharpness and readiness of our actual moral response. Because we are trained to give psychological and moral credence to the imaginary ... we may find it more difficult to identify with the real world."

Lacan was one of the survivors of what was arguably the greatest debacle in western civilization. There are people today who are cultivating visions of an even greater debacle, but this shouldn't blind us to what happened in the past. Certainly we could create a greater catastrophe than the one experienced by the world in the early forties, but it would be extremely unwise to use the vision of nuclear apocalypse to forget the dead. Is it really an accident that the antinuclear movement began in Germany in the generation that has no memory of Hitler?

As Lifton has shown in many of his works, the role of the survivor is to pay off a debt to the dead and to attempt to reestablish some sort of continuity for the living. And this reassertion of the coherence of the social structure through what Steiner might call a revitalization of the language nec- essarily passes through a stage of myth or fiction making. This is a process of symbolization through which the cata- strophic event is submitted to the symbolic order.

Thus the survivors find themselves with the task of pick- ing through the rubble, trying to salvage whatever there is to be salvaged, forging new links to hold things together. In one sense this is what Lacan was doing in his dialogue with the "luminaries" of western intellectual history. Given the historical and social context he was working in, it is hardly surprising that his own work would have the quality of being fragmented and somewhat disjointed, even fictional at times. He was not alone in adopting this mode of discourse. It corresponds in many ways to what Lévi-Strauss called *bricolage* in *La Pensée sauvage*. Bricolage is the work of a handyman, a jack-of-all-trades, someone who works with found objects, who does not have the luxury of engineering and building things according to a grand synthesis. By the end of the war Europeans had surely had enough of human engineering, efforts at creating utopian societies, new men and new women, to say nothing of the idea of selecting only the good elements and discarding those that were supposed to be bad for the society. The bricoleur works with the material at hand; he does not discard those objects that do not conform to his ideas.

Whether it is Lacan or Lévi-Strauss or Barthes or Foucault, there exists in the writings of postwar French thinkers an unmistakable poetic quality, a will to create myths and fictions, or to refashion those that had been, at least in part, discredited. Some people have found this quality annoying, and there are analysts who blithely quip that Lacan is a poet or a surrealist and not a psychoanalyst. I myself have always found such remarks mean-spirited, especially for their failure to recognize the importance of fiction making in the relationship people have with their social order and their language.

Lacan has also often been criticized for not being systematic. Clearly he never wanted to be systematic, never wanted to create a system that would inspire belief and become dogma. Within the historical context, seeing what the great intellectual systems have led to in human terms, and we would certainly have to count Marxism among them, we can at least understand why a European intellectual in the postwar period would not have been prone to systematizing. And a Freudian psychoanalyst would not have been able to overlook Freud's theory of the death drive, the drive to destruction, especially where its effects were around him every day. So Lacan could not understand why American analysts were so quick to renounce the death drive, and he was led to think that there was something about America that did not permit its people to recognize the depth of the suffering in Europe.

We are usually taught that the French and the British and the Soviets were our allies in the war, that our victory was theirs. This overlooks the fact that the United States emerged from the war as the preeminent world power. Certainly we sacrificed greatly, but from the perspective of the Europeans our sacrifices were far less than theirs. Our loss of life was less, the war never was fought on American soil, our homes and cities were not bombed, there was no combat in our streets. Moreover, the industrial matrix of the United States was not only not destroyed in the war—it was strengthened. While the Europeans were picking up the pieces, from England to Russia, the Americans were embarking on a period of prosperity, of what came to be called conspicuous consumption. These are the spoils of war, but for a people as proud as the French—limiting ourselves for the moment to Lacan's particular context—this must have rankled, especially since France came out of the war with precious little to be proud of.

One of the strangest aspects of the postwar period was the turnabout in the feelings of the French for America. When I was in France there was considerable hostility against my country and its people, and at the same time there were memories of the euphoria that overtook the country in 1944 and 1945 when the American army liberated France from the Nazi occupation. It was clear to me that Lacan had given people something to be proud of in opposing the Americans and that this gesture corresponded well to the political situation in France at the time.

I have not found a truly satisfactory explanation for the change in French attitudes toward America; perhaps there is none. Several theories have been articulated by various people and they are worth stating. The extent of the American victory in the war probably did not really become understood until the European countries had completed a little of their own rebuilding. Then they could see that America had become the leading power in the free world and that the countries of Europe were clearly located in the second rank of military, industrial, and economic powers. These once proud nations were now dependent for their defense as well as their economic recovery on the United States, and this loss of independence must have seemed a final insult. Europeans have generally considered America to be culturally inferior, second-rate, and this must have underscored the fact that the great achievements of European culture had in no way prevented the Nazi holocaust. When Europeans did look to America for intellectual leadership, they saw things like behavioral psychology or behavioral modification, which must have seemed like another form of brainwashing, or else they heard pleas for people to express their rage and anger, which could almost be called tantrum therapy. The European continent had had its fill of people expressing their hostility.

There were other reasons for the French hostility toward America. The fact that the American army saved France from Nazism was a grim reminder of the fact that the French army had barely fought for France. There was the important role played by the French resistance, but it did not capture the popular imagination to anything like the extent that films of D Day and the allied invasion did. A large part of the French population had collaborated through the formation of the government of Vichy under Pétain, and after the war any suspicion of being too friendly with an occupying army was greeted with hostility. We should remember that after the war the American army remained in France for some ten years, until De Gaulle asked it to leave, and the presence of foreign soldiers was certainly exploited by some segments of the population, particularly by the growing Communist Party that had helped organize the resistance and that had become increasingly anti-American with the development of the cold war. While most French people were no doubt euphoric about the arrival of the GIs, those who had collaborated were probably less than glad. Many people tried to forget whatever they had been doing during the occupation. And this forgetting was probably encouraged by the need to reunite the country, to repair the social fabric. We can also surmise that the French were living under a cloud of guilt for their nation's collaboration and that they dreaded American reprisals. The Russian dead are not buried in Normandy.

Where was Lacan during the war? The question has often been posed, and the answer, as far as I can tell, is that Lacan escaped from occupied France in the dead of night on a boat that took him and his wife across the Loire. For most of the occupation he was in St. Laurent-du-Var, near Antibes. Lacan's wife, Sylvia Bataille, was Jewish and, according to Catherine Clément in *Vies et légendes de Jacques Lacan*, she was denounced to the Gestapo at the beginning of the occupation. As Clément tells the story, Lacan marched into the headquarters of the Gestapo and demanded the dossier that had been compiled on his wife. Eventually he walked out with it in his hand, though Clément does not say exactly how he accomplished this, whether through bribery or force of personality. If it is true that we can tell a great deal about the character of a man by how he acts in situations of crisis, then we should recognize Lacan as a man whose personal ethical conduct was unimpeachable.

I have said that there was an unmistakably tragic quality to Lacan's role within the psychoanalytic groups in France, meaning tragic in the context of classical tragic theater. What I can add now is that, for tragedy to occur in this sense, the events befalling the hero must be bound up with his society. There is no such thing as a personal tragedy. In most cases this requirement is satisfied by the fact that the hero or heroine of the tragedy is a king or prince or general or queen.

As Lionel Trilling pointed out in "Freud and Literature," Freud's vision was essentially tragic. Thus Freudian psychoanalysis was particularly apt to account for tragic circumstances, destruction, and devastation. And yet Freud's theory was not capable of finding the way out of that tragic space, the space of the tragic theater. The popularity of psychoanalysis in France derived from the social conditions of the period after the war, and the institutes eventually were to become a theater in which social conflicts and ambiguities were dramatized, hopefully to be resolved. Lacan was taken to be a heroic figure and, however reluctantly, he played out that role. That a psychoanalyst could achieve this status publicly is not intrinsic to the psychoanalytic enterprise. If France looked to its intellectuals and artists and scientists for heroism, this was perhaps because the people upon whom a country usually calls at the end of a war, its generals and statesmen, had defaulted.

Lacan exhibited the kind of strength of character necessary for ethical heroism. When he faced down the Gestapo, when he stood by his wife and acted decisively on her behalf, he was honoring a commitment and following one of his basic principles: to keep one's word. And he held this principle not only because it makes life more livable but, more important, because he had reached the judgment that human beings are defined by language and that letting your word determine your acts is one of the essential ways we have of recognizing our debt to the dead.

The example of ethical conduct that Lacan proposed was that of Antigone. If psychoanalysis concerns ethics, then Oedipus and Hamlet, even Lear, are not the best examples of ethical action. Within the trilogy by Sophocles, *Antigone* takes us beyond Oedipus and perhaps also beyond Freud. She is one way of going beyond Freud without denying the truth of Freud's vision. Unfortunately, with her we are still within the realm of tragedy but, as I have stated, this was where Lacan was for the most part trapped. His remarks on *Antigone* were made in the seminar "The Ethics of Psychoanalysis."

The sons of Oedipus, brothers of Antigone, Eteocles and Polynices, have killed each other in battle. Eteocles was fighting on the side of the state, Thebes, and Polynices was attacking it. The ruler of Thebes, Creon, brother of Jocasta, decrees that the corpse of Eteocles be buried with full honors and that the corpse of Polynices be left to be ripped apart by dogs and birds. As Tiresias says late in the play, Creon wants to kill his enemy Polynices a second time, after he is dead. This act of supreme vengeance runs directly counter to the gods whose claim on the dead is incontrovertible, whose desire is indestructible.

Willfully disobedient, Antigone performs the proper funeral rites for her brother and will even perform them a second time. In addition, she admits openly and defiantly— Creon calls her insolent—that she has done this and that she will take responsibility. Creon sentences her to be walled up in a cave with just enough food to relieve his guilt for her death. She is condemned to be merely alive. This is untenable and, since the path of existence is barred, Antigone chooses to die; she hangs herself. As a consquence Creon's son Haemon, financé of Antigone, also kills himself, and so does Creon's wife, Eurydice. For having declared himself and the state as mightier than the gods, Creon loses everything. His loss is such that there is no possibility for it to be redeemed by love.

Antigone's action is ethical; she makes the desire of the gods into her own. She acts according to her desire, and that desire is the desire of the Other. Note that she does not pose the question of what good would accrue to her, what worldly goods will be hers. Her act is disinterested in the largest sense; she does not consider the claims of her ego for happiness. Creon, on the other hand, is a creature who represents what we are obliged to call a strong ego. He cannot tolerate a defiance of his authority, earth-bound as it may be, especially when the person who has disobeyed him is a woman. This would be for him a sign of weakness and he is strong, a representative of the power of the state. For failing to recognize the desire of the gods in the figure of a "girl," as he calls her, for failing to act according to that desire, he is punished according to the gods' justice, the *dike*, whose "unwritten law" supersedes all writs and edicts. In destroying the ego's goods, the gods dispense or pass judgment on mortals. Creon's rage against his enemy is an effort to assert the authority of the living over the laws of the dead. His is the ultimate defiance. The act of Antigone is heroic because she submits to the judgment of the gods, without procrastination.

Ultimately Antigone's desire, which Lacan said is a desire purified of any consideration of goods, is a desire for death. She acts according to that desire not because she is in love with death, as Creon asserts, but because it was decided that she will no longer be a part of the human community. In taking her own life Antigone asserts subjectively that it was not *it* that decided, but she as *I* who decided and acted on the decision. Had she procrastinated she would still have been alive, given the fact that Creon, urged by Tiresias, later decided to pardon her. Note that Antigone does not act out of despair or depression. She does not commit suicide because she cannot handle or deal with a loss of a loved one. Quite the contrary, she knows exactly what to do for a loved one who has died and, not only that, she does it. She is not in flight from responsibility and is not afraid of desire. Nor is her act one of revenge against Creon; it is not her intention that Haemon kill himself or that Creon lose everything of importance to him. About this she simply does not care. Such judgments Antigone leaves to the gods, who set their justice in motion even before she dies.

Note also that Antigone does not act out of passion. She expresses no rage, throws no tantrum. The man of passion in the play is Creon, whose passion is his revenge, but more significantly the figure of passion in her story is her father Oedipus. Here is how Lacan describes the passion of Oedipus: "man's desire, long measured, anesthetized, put to sleep by the moralists, domesticated by the educators, betrayed by the academies, very simply came to take refuge and be repressed in the most subtle and the most blind passion. As the story of Oedipus shows us, this is the passion for knowledge."

It is perhaps reasonable to suggest that the story of Antigone is an argument against precipitous action. What if she had taken time to reflect, to think things over, what if she had procrastinated before burying her brother or committing suicide? The conclusion to the play would have been more palatable and even more humane. The response must be that Antigone represents the dramatization of a principle of ethical conduct, and that this principle is not susceptible of becoming legislation for everyone. An ethical action is singular, an act of a subject, and it cannot be generalized as a set of rules that everyone can follow. It can never be written down among the laws that govern human society. And this means that one is never quite certain of the rightness or wrongness of an act when it is performed. One could even go so far as to say that pious and self-righteous moralizing, based as it is on an absolute conviction of the rightness of one's acts and the wrongness of someone else's, represents nothing more than a form of ethical cowardice.

An ethical principle can be dramatized as a tragedy, but what interests us here is how a tragedy can be transformed into a comedy or a romance—in the Shakespearean sense of the genre of romance. I have wanted to show how a Lear can become a Prospero, to show how an Antigone can become a Portia or even a Rosalind. Freud found the theme of the three caskets in *The Merchant of Venice*, and he drew a parallel between that play and *King Lear*. His essay ends precisely with the death of Lear. This is not the way I am going to conclude this book; such a conclusion would contradict the sense or direction of the story. Lacan was unequivocal about the fact that only the agency of wit or intellect could transform tragedy into comedy. If the problem faced by psychoanalysis is how to separate desire from the passion for knowledge—and to do it without reveling in the passion for ignorance—it would be a deviation to proclaim the scientificity of psychoanalysis, as much of a deviation as it would be to declare that psychoanalysts work by intuition. So in 1977 Lacan declared that, after having posed the question of the scientific status of psychoanalysis for so many years, he had come to the conclusion that it was not a science. The reason was one offered by Karl Popper, namely that psychoanalysis was "irrefutable." Lacan said that analysis was closest to rhetoric. This is consistent with his long preoccupation with the workings of language. Thus analysis seeks to persuade but not to convince, to persuade the analysand to recognize things that he knows already and to act on his desire.

The ethical imperative of psychoanalysis was stated by Freud as "Wo Es war, soll Ich werden." Clearly Lacan could not accept the standard translation, which reads "Where the id was, there the ego should be." Freud did not say *das Ich* and *das Es*; he used the pronouns without articles. Thus Lacan translated: "Where It was, there ought I to become." The transformation that ought to take place concerns the substitution of pronouns, with all the consequences that ensue. I have already alluded to this imperative in the case of Antigone. When the state, represented by Creon, determined her fate, she acted to make herself the subject of her destiny. This does not change her destiny, but it does change how she relates to it.

Let us examine a slightly less depressing instance of this

transformation. At the end of a psychoanalysis the analysand has the impression that *it* is finished, that there is nothing more to be gained from the analysis, and even that the analyst is encouraging him to terminate. With Lacan this is how *it* happened. He did not tell people, to the best of my knowledge, that they ought to terminate, that they had entered a termination phase. Often some sort of crisis erupted, usually involving the same terms that had led the analysand to consult the analyst in the first place, and this time things are different because the analysand finds himself responding differently. He no longer is willing to accept the analyst as knowing about him and no longer believes that he can acquire more knowledge from his analyst. There is nothing more to be acquired from the analyst, and it remains only to discard him, as another remnant of the past. But Lacan never accepted the idea that the analysis is ended when *it* is finished. The analysand was required to state that he as *I* was terminating and that his act was stopping the sessions for good. His deed had to be in accord with his words, and the termination phase is the period between the first statement by the analysand that he as *I* wants to terminate and the moment when he decides he will not be coming back. His desire is to terminate, he is not quitting, running off to avoid facing some difficult problem. That his deed correspond to his words, that it follow his words, reminds me of the opposite case, represented in *Waiting for Godot* when the characters at the end of the play say "Let's go" and then remain in place. Paradoxically, they do "go" because the play finishes at that moment, but their act is not ethical in the sense that Antigone's is.

Antigone was not an intellectual; nor does she act out of instinct or emotion. There is great intelligence involved in her judgment and subsequent action. What Antigone does not do is intellectualize—she does not ponder the rightness or wrongness of her act either before or after it; she does not deploy her mind to procrastinate about something she knows she must do; nor does she indulge in post-mortem guilt over whether she should or should not have done it. Intellectualization, if it means anything, is a perversion of the mind in the service of the ego. More commonly it is called rationalization—for a failure to act or for a mistaken act.

Lacan was an intellectual, but he certainly never intellectualized, in this sense of the word. To engage in the process, which is as ponderous and cumbersome as the word itself, you must have time, a good deal of time. Intellectualization is intimately related to procrastination. It implies a will to explain away things, to interpret them to death, to concoct an endless series of reasons telling why and wherefore and leaving the deed undone. Or else, if the deed has been done, the rationalizations declare that the ego wishes to undo it, wishes that it had never happened.

Not only did Lacan not intellectualize; he did not encourage or promote the use of this defense in others. He did this in a very simple way, by never giving you the time to intellectualize. There is no way to intellectualize within the frame of the short session. This is not to say that analysands did not try, but given the fact that such rationalization was generally not receivable by Lacan, the analysand eventually was obliged to give it up, discovering in the process why he was drawn to the habit.

Labeling intellectualization a defense does not make all uses of the intellect suspect. Quite the contrary. Lacan encouraged the workings of the intellect, of wit, and of the characteristic that was most indicative of its workings— brevity. The mode of the intellect tends toward the aphoristic. Brevity, we know, is the soul of wit, and equivocation is its body. Why equivocation? Because any rational explanation, any explanation that carries a meaning that can be grasped by the ego, tends to feed a self-image that does nothing to threaten the ego's identity. And this identity, being defined in terms of life, wishes to have nothing to do with death or the dead, thus with action or desire.

By all accounts Antigone was lacking in wit, in cunning, in guile. Not wanting to place blame, we say that extraordinary social situations sometimes cast these qualities in a light that makes them difficult to recognize. If psychoanalysis is related most closely to rhetoric, then certainly wit, cunning, and guile are essential to its practice. The finest therapeutic example I have come across is from Shakespeare's *As You Like It*. Orlando, the protagonist, is suffering from a common malady—he is in love, passionately. He wanders through the forest of Arden in search of his beloved Rosalind, writing sickening love poems and tacking them on to trees. Rosalind is also in the forest, disguised as Ganymede, the disguise assuring her safe passage. Since, as Lacan said, true love is always reciprocal, she is in love with Orlando. This sets the scene for their meeting in Act III.

In this encounter Orlando, blinded by love, does not recognize Rosalind, but she recognizes him. She does not, however, remove her mask, announce her identity, and requite his passion. Instead she tells him that being in love is a sickness and that she can cure this sickness through counsel. She even encourages him to come to see her every day to effect a cure. She proposes playing the role of Rosalind to permit him to get over his love.

But why does she not simply respond to his demand for love? Wouldn't that have been more natural and more human? The reason, I suggest, is that she has sufficient wit about her to know what she desires and also to know that Orlando, in his present state, is in no position to give her what she wants. Her response to passion, as she describes it, is "for every passion something and for no passion truly anything."

And so in Act IV the treatment begins, and Orlando presses his suit on Rosalind disguised as Ganymede pretending to be Rosalind. She says that she refuses his suit, that she does not want him, to which Orlando responds that he will die. Here Rosalind intervenes to propose that if death is what is wanted then Orlando should die "by attorney," that is, by proxy, through a representative. No one has ever died for love "in his own person." She concludes her speech with the famous line: "Men have died from time to time, and worms have eaten them, but not for love."

We assume that Rosalind does not really mean it, since we know that she is in love, and yet, since we know that the statement is uttered by a dramatic character, through a mask, then what this means is that she really does mean it. So what is she saying? First, that dying is not an act of love, is not a proof of love, whether it be done by Orlando or Socrates or Lacan. And worms eat corpses, not for love but because of their appetite. I don't think this means that death is natural, but rather that death has an appetite for the living. People die because it is death's desire, and for no other reason. Note that Rosalind does not deny or denigrate the desire for death. What she says is that it is not an act of love, on the one hand, and on the other that it can be negotiated through a proxy. In our terms, it can be negotiated through a signifier. As Lacan pointed out in "The Ethics of Psychoanalysis," the difference between tragedy and comedy is the presence in the latter of the phallus, as privileged signifier. Perhaps he was thinking of *Lysistrata*, but the phallic references in Shakespeare's high comedies would have done as well.

The example he used to close the seminar was from *The Merchant of Venice*. He chose the story of the pound of flesh and the way it was negotiated by Portia. This was the part of the play that Freud neglected to mention in "The Theme of the Three Caskets." Perhaps the reason was the figure of Shylock, the Jewish usurer who poses the problem of antisemitism in European civilization. Through Shylock, the Jew is posed as Other, as capital Other, as foreign to the values of Christian culture and religion. Shylock is also defined as desiring; as greedy, envious, bound to a lust for flesh. While it is not explicit in Shakespeare's play, the figure of the Jew was often associated with insatiable lust. As Gratiano says to Shylock: "thy desires are wolvish, bloody, starved, and ravenous." The idea of bloodlust may very well be a reference to the strange and dark ritual of circumcision. The ritual cutting of the body may even remind us of the cutting of the session as practiced by Lacan. In both cases the cut is symbolic as well as real. Interestingly, most of the things Lacan was berated and condemned for, his place as Other, are characteristics that have been associated with social groups or races thought to be Other.

The moral condemnation of Otherness is racist; of this there is little doubt. The elimination of difference was seen at times to be essential to the creation of an ideal state, a state in which sameness is the order of the day, where everyone should be like "me," like "my Self." So when Lacan refused to create a theory of the Self, when he proposed an ethic that resides on the Other's desire, when he theorized about the topology of the cut and the mark, when he emphasized the Law and the Letter and the Pact, he was firmly sustaining a cultural tradition that was central to Freud and that Lacan's own cultural tradition had tried on numerous occasions to repress. Isn't this what he really meant when he called for a return to Freud—not addressed to the IPA, but to the French nation?

This is not to say that Lacan's theory of psychoanalysis is simply a political allegory. Political acts and activities are one response to the basic structure of human existence, but certainly not the only one that is ethical. And I think we would all agree that racism does not merely victimize the Other. Those who attempt to erase cultural difference, who wish to create a society in which Otherness is nonexistent, come to be alienated from their own desire, since this desire is the desire of the Other. Significantly, the philosophical movement of existentialism that was so popular in Europe after the war addressed precisely these issues, though in a way that Lacan could not accept. What he could not accept was the bleak pessimism, the faith and trust in self-consciousness, the search for liberty within a situation of enslavement, the denial of the efficacy of action. (These points are specifically made in his paper on the mirror stage.) He also criticized existentialism for the idealization of the sexual act, an idealization he criticized because it tends to see sex as an act of love, an act that erases difference. Taking the sex act as an ideal, Lacan said, was "voyeuristic-sadistic." The same should be said about the current idealization of "relating."

For the most part, however, Lacan did not address the historical implications of these theoretical issues. We are surprised to find in his work no references to the neurotic problems faced by those who had survived the war. The emphasis I have placed on the role of the dead in the affairs of the living is not something that Lacan discussed explicitly. And yet is it too much to think that the presence of ghosts of those destroyed in the war was a significant element in the mental life of the survivors? I remember once at a seminar Lacan said that his writing style, his enigmatic way of expressing himself, was necessitated by the fact that if he had spoken otherwise, "they" would not have let him speak. I remember wondering what on earth he was talking about. Certainly sexuality had long since become a fact of life in western countries; no one was likely to be shocked by sexual innuendo or references. But perhaps he was thinking of the dead, of the ghosts that continued to haunt the minds of the survivors. Perhaps Lacan thought that the history of his country and his civilization in this century was simply too much to grapple with directly. Doubtless he knew that the best way to think the unthinkable was first to empty it of all content. Only later, once the structures of discourse and society are reestablished, can the forbidden and forbidding contents be replaced.

The resolution of the problem of Shylock proposed by Shakespeare is untenable. What happens in *The Merchant of Venice* is that Portia resolves the dispute over the pound of flesh by telling Shylock—Portia is disgused as a doctor of laws—that he may take the pound of flesh but that he may not shed any blood. She then says that his desire for his due, for what is owed him under the contract he made with Antonio, is an intent to murder that can only be expunged by his converting to Christianity. On the one hand we may say that Portia declares that the pound of flesh is a symbol and not a reality, but, on the other, the conversion of Shylock to Christianity can only be read as a refusal to recognize otherness, a refusal to recognize the desire of the Other.

Within the context of this book, the story of Shylock can be read another way. Shylock, as Other, is one from whom something has been stolen—his daughter Jessica has been stolen, along with a certain amount of money. And the pound of flesh, which I have read with a distinctly phallic cast, is a signifier that Shylock is shown to want to have for real. Shylock's conversion is not the reassertion of the primacy of the symbolic; quite the contrary, it circumvents the real to show the triumph of life and love in the imaginary. What is intolerable about Shylock is his representing the fact that the gods will ultimately get their pound of flesh for real, and that this flesh will not be redeemed.

The problem facing the postwar generation in Europe was not so much how to assimilate Otherness, how to integrate it, but rather how to reconstruct western ethics, to transform the traditional way of approaching the questions of metaphysics and theology. The subversion of the concept of subjectivity that had informed western thought was the first part of this project. The second was the establishment of a dialogue or a dialectic with Otherness. There was obviously something wrong with the foundation of civilization, and it was no longer possible to continue as if nothing had happened.

Lacan conceptualized this project in such a way as to reject the solutions or paths of increased self-consciousness. He refused to call upon the consciousness that had produced the holocaust and ask it to minister to the survivors. He would not require consciousness to show itself strong enough to integrate the madness it itself had unleashed. To make the experience of the Second World War into an object of consciousness would have been the ultimate insult for those who had perished—ultimate insult because it would have made that experience into food for consciousness, an occasion or challenge against which consciousness could show again its strength, its ability to assert itself as being alive in the face of the most horrifying realities. That consciousness implies the triumph of life in face of adversity, and that its triumph can only be at the expense of a scapegoat, this was one of the truths that emerged in Europe after the war.

The historical juncture at which Lacan lived and worked imposed certain demands and determined the course of things for him as it did for others. It also had a good deal to do with how he heard the discourse of other analysts, particularly American analysts. To have given American analysts almost a demonic role was not to Lacan's credit. But this does not obviate the fact that American analysts ought to reexamine their theoretical presuppositions in the light of Lacan's critique.

Let me shift gears for a moment to introduce a story, a myth, that provides a fictional account of the construction of something out of a holocaust. The story is of a survivor, of one who lived to tell the tale, of the best-known survivor of the destruction of Troy, Aeneas. The fact that the founding of Rome should be the consequence of the Trojan War, which itself began with a mythic event called the Judgment of Paris, should alert us to the parallel between this story and Lacan's career. I cannot guarantee that Lacan saw this parallel, though he did deliver the speech "Function and Field of Speech and Language" in Rome and he was a man well versed in the classics. If there is a connection it would explain why Lacan put such great importance in the founding of his school and perhaps also why, when the Ecole freudienne was dissolved and the dissidents were put out, Lacan invoked the statement of Cato the Elder in declaring: *Delenda est Carthago* (Carthage must be destroyed). And I would also doubt that Lacan with his interest in language and naming would have ignored Paris, the man for whom his city was named.

Paris, the man, was the son of Priam, king of Troy. He was called upon by Zeus to decide a dispute among three goddesses, Hera, queen of the gods, Athena, goddess of war, and Aphrodite, goddess of beauty. Paris was asked to decide which was the fairest. Hera spoke first and promised Paris an empire if he chose her. Athena spoke second and promised victory in battle. The third, Aphrodite, disrobed and told Paris that if he chose her she would give him the most beautiful woman in the world. He chose the third and his prize was Helen, wife of Menelaus. The theft of Helen led, of course, to the Trojan War and the destruction of the city of Troy. One might say that Paris and his city suffered the wrath of the two scorned matriarchs.

That Aeneas went on to found Rome instead of staying in Carthage with his love, Queen Dido, indicates that personal happiness must take second place to an ethical responsibility, to a destiny. It is clear that Lacan felt when he dissolved the Ecole that too many of his followers had remained in Carthage, that they had opted for personal rewards and had turned their backs on the historical and mythical implications of their practice. It is difficult to blame those who make such a decision—what after all do we have against those who want simply to be happy and normal?—but Lacan could not accept this sort of abrogation of responsibility, this failure to see that one's act as a psychoanalyst is more than a good way to make a living and to have a nice life. Lacan was not a humanist, to say the least.

For Aeneas, Carthage was a *lieu de passage*. It was the place where he told the story of the destruction of Troy, and it was through his telling that he came to seduce Dido. For the Ecole freudienne Lacan wanted "the pass" to be a similar *lieu de passage*, but as sometimes happens with these things, the pass became the thing itself. It became an end for too many people, an excuse to stop trying to advance psychoanalysis. Practice, in other words, had become too comfortable, easy, successful; no one felt the need to continue to question and debate. This happens in other groups of psychoanalysts, and when it does the theory becomes stale and musty; it repeats the same questions and the old answers, thereby losing the excitement and spark that had led people to psychoanalysis in the first place. Too concerned with guarding the flame, refusing to repeat the act of theft that acquired fire in the first place, psychoanalysts have a tendency to let the fire go out, to turn their theory into dogma, their training rituals into the cut and dried absorption of a certain orthodoxy in conformity to the opinions of those who retain power in the institutes. It was not so much that Lacan was against happiness as that he saw a bourgeois complacency creeping into the analytic group in Paris, with insidious consequences for theory and for practice.

At the end of an analysis the analysand is, like Aeneas, a survivor. He has survived the destruction of his narcissism, especially insofar as that narcissism had invested the analysis itself. This is one way of reading the destruction of Troy; it differs from the modern holocaust, which represents an insane attempt to assert the hegemony of narcissism, identified with a state and a race.

What precipitates the end of the analysis is a ruse, of which I cannot think of a better example than the Trojan horse, monument to the guile and cunning of Odysseus. According to Aeneas the Trojans accepted the horse as an offering because they were led to believe first that refusal to accept it would mean the destruction of their empire and, second, because they believed that it would make them invincible in battle. The horse represents the promise of life, of eternal life, prosperity, victory—the triumph of narcissism and the defeat of death.

Like the Trojan War, psychoanalysis can often become a seemingly endless standoff between two competing forces. It ends when the analysand thinks that psychoanalysis is life itself, when he feels that the analysis has guaranteed him eternal life in the future. In some cases the analysand feels that, when he terminates, the next step is some kind of immortality for himself; in others he feels that he will become someone who can confer eternal life on others. It is precisely these illusions that the termination of the analysis dissipates.

But that is not the end. Lacan placed great emphasis on the pass, on the analysand's telling his story after his analysis is over. It would seem that the analysand retains a wish, that after all the effort and sacrifice, after giving up or even being cheated out of his narcissistic attachments, he will gain something that we may call an eternal reward, a pot of gold at the end of the rainbow. However well analyzed he is, he will continue to cherish the hope that one day the queen of Carthage will fall into his arms. If telling his story feeds this last illusion, the one the analysis cannot treat when it becomes a reality after the analysis, then the immolation of Dido, the immolation of a mirage, is the consequence of his having made the judgment to sacrifice wealth, happiness, and the queen of Carthage to continue on his path, to do what his destiny dictates.

If Lacan was following the script of the *Aeneid*, then his 1953 discourse in Rome ("Function and Field") corresponds to the victory of Aeneas over his enemy Turnus.

Lacan's enemy was the school of ego psychology he found occupying the Freudian field. But Lacan never seemed to accept his victory; he was always looking over his shoulder to intercept whoever might steal the spoils he had won. This man who asserted the primacy of desire was tremendously demanding, to the end. He wanted respect and recognition but was never satisfied when he obtained them. He still demanded love—at best he gave this drama the dignity of tragedy. Perhaps the spirit of the times imposed this role on him; Freudian psychoanalysis did not provide him with the conceptual tools to negotiate it. To his credit, perhaps, he did not blame Freud. He directed his wrath at Freudians, at those who did not have the courage to reformulate psychoanalysis in a direction Freud had not foreseen.

Lacan once said that he had given his life to psychoanalysis. Psychoanalysis has surely profited from the exchange. But his flaw was that he saw no limits to this service and did not recognize that this was not what analysis wanted of him. In the person of its practitioners, psychoanalysis did not realize what was behind his words: "Je te demande de refuser ce que je t'offre, parce que ce n'est pas ça" (I ask you to refuse what I offer you, because that's not it).

For my part I have told the story that I experienced. Perhaps it is symptomatic that a grasp of Lacan's theory is best attained in conjunction with a sense of the man himself. For this man was never quite as Other as he wished. His "saying"—when, where, and how he said what he had to say—can never be accounted for by a written text. It can only be circumscribed. That the saying of one man becomes an event, transforming the discourse that sustains the existence of those around him, this is intolerable for any human being.

Jacques Lacan saw himself as a solitary figure. He placed his work in direct opposition to the ideological bias toward life, toward being, toward the flowing of an essential humanity.

The man was out of touch and out of step with the body of opinion that ravaged the discourse of his time. Clearly he saw no other way.

Not one to daydream about actualizing human possibilities, Lacan defined psychoanalytic practice as a repeated encounter with the impossible. And he located that practice under the figure of the knot. The impossibility of psychoanalysis, first noted by Freud, is not a counsel of despair. Quite the contrary. Precisely because it is impossible, psychoanalysis produces results, lets things happen outside itself, lets people exist.

Of Lacan's passage I inscribe these notes in haste. It takes time to pursue a psychoanalysis, but only a moment as I conclude.